BODILY ALTERATIONS

Wisslon

For Betty & Bob —
Two very dear friends —
With love,
    Wendy Seymour
       Dec. 1990.

Studies in Society

Titles include:

The Migrant Presence Martin
Race, Class and Rebellion in the South Pacific Mamak and Ali
Children and Families in Australia Burns and Goodnow
Johnsonville Pearson
Australian Community Studies and Beyond Wild
Open Cut Williams
The Ethnic Dimension Martin and Encel
The Aging Experience Russell
Australian Cinema Tulloch
Strikes in Australia Waters
Class Consciousness in Australia Chamberlain
Heathcote Wild
Practice and Belief Black and Glasner
Law, Capitalism and Democracy O'Malley
Eclipse of Equality Pearson and Thorns
The Family in the Modern World Burns, Jools and Bottomley
Women, Social Welfare and the State Baldock and Cass
Ideology of Motherhood Wearing
Indians in a White Australia de Lepervanche
Confronting School and Work Dwyer, Wilson and Woock
Ethnicity, Class and Gender in Australia Bottomley and de Lepervanche
The Faith of Australians Mol
Social Theory and the Australian City Kilmartin, Thorns and Burke
The First Wave Lewins and Ly
Surveys in Social Research de Vaus
Australian Ways Manderson
Custody and Control Asher
Where it Hurts Russell and Schofield
Caring for Australia's Children Brennan and O'Donnell
Shaping Futures Wilson and Wyn
Health Care Issues Bates and Linder-Pelz
Blue, White and Pink Collar Workers in Australia Williams
The Gender Agenda Evans
Regulation and Repression Edwards
For Freedom and Dignity Metcalfe
Technology and the Labour Process Willis
Australian Attitudes Kelley and Bean
Medical Dominance Willis

BODILY ALTERATIONS

An introduction to a sociology of the body for health workers

Wendy Seymour

ALLEN & UNWIN
Sydney Wellington London Boston

© Wendy Seymour 1989
This book is copyright under the Berne Convention.
No reproduction without permission. All rights reserved.

First published in 1989
Allen & Unwin Australia Pty Ltd
An Unwin Hyman Company
8 Napier Street, North Sydney, NSW 2059 Australia

Allen & Unwin New Zealand Limited
75 Ghuznee Street, Wellington, New Zealand

Unwin Hyman Limited
15–17 Broadwick Street, London W1V 1FP England

Unwin Hyman Inc.
8 Winchester Place, Winchester, Mass 01890 USA

National Library of Australia
Cataloguing-in-Publication Entry:

Seymour, Wendy.
  Bodily alterations: an introduction to a sociology of
  the body for health workers.

  Bibliography.
  Includes index.
  ISBN 0 04 374009 X.

  1. Rehabilitation. 2. Social medicine.
  3. Paraplegics—Rehabilitation. 4. Quadriplegics—Rehabilitation.
  I. Title.

362.4'04

Library of Congress Catalog Number: 89–084873

Set in 10.5/12pt English Times by Graphicraft Typesetters, Hong Kong
Produced by SRM Production Services Sdn Bhd, Malaysia

Contents

Acknowledgements		vi
Glossary		vii
Preface		ix
1	Listening to the patient	1
2	The body and its activities	11
3	Health and illhealth	24
4	What is disease?	38
5	Rehabilitation—the challenge to medicine	52
6	Person to paralysed patient	66
7	Paralysed patient to person	84
8	Barriers to transformation	97
9	What is health after disease or trauma?	108
10	Rehabilitation—the dilemmas	126
Bibliography		137
Index		141

Acknowledgements

I thank all the quadriplegic and paraplegic people who, in acting as my informants, contributed to this book. Their perceptive insights into their own condition provided me with the information for this study; but, in a very real sense, they wrote it.

The director, the late Dr G. Nambiar, and the staff of the Spinal Injuries Unit of the Royal Adelaide Hospital extended to me, an inquisitive outsider, courtesy, friendliness and help.

The provocative ideas of Bruce Kapferer and Michael Muetzelfeldt have stimulated my thoughts in ways that they will recognise many times in the following pages. Betty Yeatman read the final draft and offered invaluable comments and criticisms.

I thank Rachela Lombardi, Marie Abbott, Dianne Feutrill, Rosanna Sorace and Val Riddiford at the South Australian Institute of Technology for their important contributions in typing the manuscript.

Glossary

Afferent pathways: nerves proceeding toward the spinal cord
Anorexia: lack or loss of appetite
Anorexia nervosa: a psychological condition characterised by a prolonged refusal to eat, resulting in emaciation, amenorrhea, disturbance concerning body image and an abnormal fear of becoming obese
Bulimia nervosa: a variant of anorexia nervosa. Characterised by overpowering urge to eat large amounts of food followed by induced vomiting or abuse of laxatives to avoid any gain of weight
Cachexia: a general wasting of the body during a chronic disease
Catheter: a hollow, flexible tube that can be inserted into a vessel or cavity of the body to withdraw or instil fluids
Catheterisation: in this study refers to the insertion of a catheter into the bladder through the urethra for the relief of urinary retention
Contracture: permanent shortening of a muscle or of fibrous tissue causing an abnormal position of a joint
Decubitus ulcer: inflammation, sore or ulcer in the skin over a bony prominence resulting from prolonged pressure on the part of the body
Efferent pathways: nerves directed away from the spinal cord
Electrolyte balance: the equilibrium between the chemical composition of bodily fluids
Iatrogenic: a condition caused by treatment or diagnostic procedures
Involuntary muscle: also called smooth or unstriated muscle. The muscle of such organs as intestines, stomach and other viscera, not under conscious or voluntary control
Tracheostomy: an opening cut through the neck into the trachea to facilitate breathing

viii Bodily alterations

Ryles tube: a feeding tube passing through the nose to the stomach
Respirator: an apparatus used to improve ventilation of the lungs
Urinary drainage: in these situations, drainage of urine from the bladder through the catheter
Vasomotor control: relating to the nerves which supply the muscles that control the internal diameter of the blood vessels

Preface

The sudden loss of body function or control is a calamitous event. Quadriplegia and paraplegia most often occur in young people with most of their lives before them. By asking how people restructure their identities after severe body loss, this book presents an introduction to a sociology of the body. Although the insights raised by this work will have direct relevance for students of health-related disciplines and workers in rehabilitation settings, the material will also relate to many other situations in which people experience a change from one state to another—situations such as migration, job loss and divorce. As well as these applied contexts, the book will stand on its own as a sociological exploration of the relationship between the body, the self and society.

A thorough theoretical framework underpins the work. The study asserts the centrality of the body in identity construction. The body is the showcase of the self, the core of all understanding about oneself and the society in which one lives. The disruption of self-identity caused by the sudden and severe body alterations of quadriplegia and paraplegia present a rare opportunity to observe the separation of the body and the self. Exploration of the deconstruction and subsequent reconstitution of self-identity through the understandings of people who have experienced permanent body paralysis provide critical insights into the relationship between the body, the self and society in many other contexts, and in a more general analytical sense.

Medical sociology and anthropology are rapidly expanding fields, both in their own right, but also as the undergraduate and post-graduate education of health professionals moves away from the more didactic orientations of medicine itself. I feel strongly that this work will fill an important gap in a large and rapidly expanding field of tertiary education. Health workers are, after all, body workers par excellence.

1 Listening to the patient

Can you imagine never walking again? Never again leaping from your bed on a sunny morning to search for the daily paper under the car before settling down with coffee and toast to catch up on the world outside? Strolling around shopping arcades choosing clothes for a special occasion, or maybe some food to share with friends? Stopping off on the way home to visit friends, sharing your treats with them on their balcony overlooking the surf?

A life spent in a wheelchair may not sound so bad to some people. But try to imagine never standing again, never rising from your chair to greet a friend, your eyes set perpetually at the level of other people's waists. Can you conceive how you would manage your life if you could not weed the garden, paint the roof, change a light globe or ride a bus?

Consider the most routine tasks of daily life—to wash, dress and feed yourself. Not only may you be unable to perform these tasks, but you may have to ask others to perform these most intimate tasks for you. Not only can you no longer reach out to hug your child, but you cannot feel her arms around you. You may even be incapable of lifting a glass of water to your mouth, turning the page of a book, or brushing away a fly.

Such disabilities are almost impossible for healthy people to imagine. Movement, sensation, and normal bodily functions are taken for granted, fundamental elements of every situation.

Yet these are the issues that paralysed people must face. The sudden disruption of movement and control in a previously well functioning body is a calamitous event. But the physical loss also involves an infringement of a person's self-understanding. The body has become, in effect, separated from the identity of the paralysed person. The reality of the physical loss is unequivocal. The conceptual understanding of that reality is not so clear. The latter is of course consequent upon the former, but the two are by no means convergent in time, space or level of understanding. The physical body is no longer appropriate to the concept of self. Readjustment of the discrepancy between former understanding and the new physical reality, the focus of this book, is most often a long and difficult process.

In this book I examine the consequences of this rupture through the understanding of people who have become paralysed as a result of injury or infection. Quadriplegia and paraplegia are not diseases in their own right. Quadriplegia and paraplegia are the consequence—disabilities that occur as a result of trauma or an infective organism. Although this particular medical syndrome illustrates a sudden and dramatic infringement of a person's self-concept, many who suffer from it are able to reintegrate totally into society, and to enjoy full and satisfying social relationships. Their paralysed limbs can never be forgotten, but in such cases these serious physical limitations are able to be incorporated into a reconstituted healthy self. The reconstituted self accommodates quite different elements from the former self.

The problems experienced by paralysed people demand examination in their own right. But these substantive issues provoke more general questions about the relationship between the individual and society. What is the relationship of the body to the self? What part does the body play in social interaction? Is there a relationship between the body and society? The issues of direct concern to paralysed people have wide sociological implications. Extensive body paralysis presents a rare opportunity to observe a separation of the body from the self. The body is no longer integral to the self. Future actions based on past experience and meaning can be assumed no more.

This study explores the manner in which the relationship between the body and self-identity is altered by trauma or disease. The physical, social and personal losses experienced by people who have become quadriplegics or paraplegics provide a model by which we may analyse the losses experienced by other people with different medical or social conditions that also challenge self-identity. The sequential exploration of the deconstruction of self (in chapter 6) and its reconstruction (in chapter 7) in relation to quadriplegia and paraplegia provides an obvious, dramatic and highly visible example of the same processes that occur in many other diseases, illnesses and syndromes.

A heart attack, although not involving the massive physical losses associated with quadriplegia and paraplegia, can provoke extreme grief. Even in these days of open heart surgery and heart transplantation, this organ is still shrouded in mystery, symbolism and fear. The heart of the matter is the central, essential part of an argument, just as the heart is the essential organ for life. The soul is thought to reside in the heart. Having killed an enemy, to then cut out his heart was seen as the ultimate act of revenge. To cut out a man's heart was to discard his soul—to separate his soul from his body—and to condemn his body to eternal isolation and damnation.

The intricate mysteries associated with the heart would seldom be addressed in a modern coronary disease unit, yet the meaning of a myocardial infarction to the person who experiences such a catastrophe may still involve hidden emotions and reactions that have important implications for rehabilitation—for the reconstitution of self-identity.

The progressive losses associated with inflammatory arthritis may seem less dramatic. Although the physical loss is unlikely to be sudden, the ongoing necessity to reconstruct self-image to be consistent with the person's continually deteriorating body function makes this condition extremely difficult to cope with. Many other conditions involve a similar slow but inexorable deterioration of motor function and body appearance, and are also particularly difficult for the person involved.

Loss of a part of the body, an amputation, can present another vivid example of the separation of body and self-image. Although many logical medical explanations exist for phantom limb sensations, such sensations may, in part, relate to the lack of realignment of self-image with the new body state.

The breast, like the heart, is embedded in symbolism and social meaning. To be a woman is to have breasts. The task of reconstitution of self as a woman, as a sexual being, as a mother, after a mastectomy can be a formidable task in the face of the strong social attitudes associated with this organ.

Additions to the body, as well as amputations, may also seriously challenge self-image. A colostomy bag, a breast reconstruction, joint replacements and, particularly, facial reconstruction may involve severe disjunction between self-image and new body form.

Ageing brings with it inevitable losses, which are often identified but seldom analysed. Again, the continual necessity to reconcile bodily changes such as greying hair and wrinkling skin with a self-image constructed in earlier times is a difficult task. With the discriminatory attitudes about old people in our society, the positive attitude of someone who looks old but feels young is most likely to be short lived. Strong social pressures from many sources are most often successful in forcing a reconciliation of

4 Bodily alterations

body and self-image—to the great detriment of many older people.

Alterations in the relationship between body and self-identity in the extreme situations exemplified by quadriplegia and paraplegia give valuable insights into the interaction between the body and identity in these and many other less permanent conditions with which people must come to terms. More generally, events involving a change in status, such as marriage, divorce, childbirth, financial loss, migration and unemployment, are also susceptible to some of the analytical understandings arising out of this research.

My field work sample is small. I acknowledge the diversity of conditions causing the severe motor and sensory paralyses which are the subject of my primary investigations. Of the medical processes involved, I claim no more than the most basic understanding. The same medical syndrome affects each individual differently. Not only is there great variety in the level of the lesion in a traumatic injury, but the initial severity and the degree of recovery from an infection such as paralytic poliomyelitis is diverse. The damage experienced by my informants in this study represents the severe end of the spectrum. Their losses are functionally similar to the losses experienced by traumatic quadriplegics and paraplegics, and in this study these conditions will be treated as one.

However, while sensitive to my limited medical knowledge, I submit that this is not of paramount importance to this study. I have gathered information about a group of people who have experienced roughly the same type of interruption to their lives. They have been forced to reorder their understanding of themselves in relation to a broad set of common experiences. Some of these people were injured twenty years ago, others much more recently. Several of these people spent months in a respirator to sustain their lives after poliomyelitis. Others were never in danger of losing their lives after the initial traumatic injury, but have spent many years reconciling an impetuous dive into shallow water, a corner taken too sharply in a car, or the negligence of others with the bodily state in which they now find themselves.

I have talked to people in a wide range of age and social groups and medical categories. I do not wish to impose an artificial gloss of consistency or unity on the people whom I have chosen to illustrate my hypothesis. But my paramount interest in this study is people, not medical entities; the meaning of their experiences for them, not the clinical facts. The people I have talked to have experienced a broad set of structural and processual similarities. Each of these factors will influence the reconstitution of the person after the event, but none has objective or predictive reality because the experiences of each person are unique. One person's experience is different from that of another, despite the fact that both pass through a superficially similar set of physical circumstances and situations. I justify my selection of data on these grounds.

I intended, initially, to confine my field research to quadriplegic and paraplegic people in the community, without reference to specific institutional collectivities of such people.

I was introduced to two respondents by a friend. These two people, Bob and Pam, are well known spokespeople for quadriplegics and paraplegics, although each from a different position. Pam introduced me to Phillip and Michael, not friends of hers, but known to her through association with paraplegic sport.

Bob introduced me to Tony. Sudden injury to a formerly healthy self is an important element in my study. Tony's physical loss, although profound, was not of sudden onset. For this reason I have excluded this informant, although his perceptive insights into his own condition have given me valuable clues in seeking information from others.

Tony introduced me to Frank. These two men live permanently in an institution, although not an institution oriented specifically to paralysed people. They see each other occasionally, but are not close friends. Jim and Maggie were shadows from my past. I remembered these two people as poliomyelitis patients in an acute infectious diseases hospital where I had worked as a physiotherapist. I had seen neither of them in the intervening years nor did I know what had happened to them. To meet these two people again, and to hear how they had reconstituted their lives, was a special delight.

I am taking care to discuss the selection of my informants. Some of the information these people have given me seems quite extraordinary. I do not want to suggest that what these people have told me is typical. But I do want to emphasise that to my knowledge my seven major informants are not representative of a single age, sex or social group, nor do they hold a united political position.

The 'randomness' of any research selection is always problematic. A chain of selection can develop when one informant perceives the issues that concern the questioner and refers the questioner to another informant whom she or he feels will fulfill these expectations.

I do not consider that this has occurred to any extent in my collection of data. I emphasise, however, that this exploration is not a statistical survey. My aim is to expose possibilities, not generalities; to challenge everyday assumptions about the disruptive effects of disease and trauma on body image.

As I said, I intended to confine my research to people in the community, but as I listened to my informants, I realised that the time spent in an institution was very influential for each of them. Hospital care is inevitable for all paralysed people, followed by a period of rehabilitation. It is within the context of the institution that a person may come to understand him or herself as a paralysed patient, that meaning is given to experience. Although the period spent in the hospital and rehabilitation unit is only a short time in a person's overall progress from illhealth to health again, it is an extremely influential time and must be explored.

For this reason, I became a participant observer at a spinal rehabilitation unit over a period of three months. I was free to question staff and patients. I participated in barbecues, shopping excursions, card games, and much general conversation. I joined staff conferences, took tea and lunch with different staff members, attended physiotherapy and occupational therapy sessions, and observed gymnasium and hydrotherapy programmes.

Conversations with my seven main informants were lengthy and detailed. Discussions with some of these informants took place over several weeks, and amounted to many hours of specific information. At the spinal unit, however, my data collection was more casual. I specifically did not collect information from these people in the same way as I had done for my informants outside the institution. Their recent loss and location within an institution made me sensitive to their vulnerability. For this reason I avoided long or detailed face to face conversations with these people, and I have not specifically identified them, even with a pseudonym, in this text.

Nevertheless, my time at this institution provided invaluable insights into the process of becoming a patient. The information given to me in casual conversation by paralysed people in the institution was crucial for this study. To observe at first hand the many institutional processes that make up the medical reality was vital to my understanding of the information given to me by my original informants outside the institution.

While quadriplegia and paraplegia are not rare, these conditions are sufficiently uncommon for quadriplegics and paraplegics to be readily identifiable. There are enough broad points of identification amongst people who are, and people who interact with, quadriplegic and paraplegic people to make anonymity important. I have, of course, changed the names of all my informants. Rather than presenting my data in the form of case studies, which would perhaps be easier for the reader to follow, I have deliberately broken up the data and dispersed it throughout the study. I hope that the inconvenience that this may cause the reader can be excused by my overriding desire to preserve the anonymity of my informants.

My commitment to anthropological and sociological methods and theories will be obvious throughout. My aim is not to select and present empirical examples in order to prove the superiority of a particular theory, but to use aspects of several theoretical perspectives to illuminate the experiences of people whose self-image has been challenged. The information given to me by my respondents is, of course, sufficient in its own right; a theoretical analysis will not change the experiences for these people. But by exploring the data with analytical tools we may increase our awareness of the social processes influencing these experiences. Such knowledge will form the basis for change—change that may avert or alleviate some of the destructive aspects of these processes for other people with different conditions whose self-image is similarly challenged. The salient features of the perspectives you will find in this study are outlined here, but will be developed more fully as the study evolves.

The retrospective construction of biography is a difficult exercise for all concerned. What constitutes data is an explanation of the meaning of an event after the event has happened. The past is interpreted from the vantage point of the present. Alfred Schutz's discussion of 'because motives' illuminates this problem, and will be discussed more fully later (Schutz, 1972:86ff). In order to look back on what has gone before, one must deal in because motives. This is quite honest and legitimate. But the issues from the past that a person selects as relevant are determined by his or her present interests. Present interests depend on a sedimentation of knowledge, experience and meaning over many years.

I, the information gatherer, also see the informant as he or she now is. I decide the importance of the information given me from the position in which we now both find ourselves. What I present as data is an interpretation of an interpretation. Time and social situation have changed, and so has the meaning of the event. An important prerequisite for understanding the data presented here is an awareness of the emergent and processual nature of the constitution of what comes to be called data.

I defer to two main theoretical paradigms in the exploration of my field research: social phenomenology and symbolic interactionism. I intend as much as possible to maintain the integrity of the people I study. The social world is however, largely taken for granted by its inhabitants. Within the 'natural attitude' the individual unquestionably accepts his or her world (Natanson, 1973:228). Substantial cognitive structures are built on unexamined assumptions: 'everyone knows'; 'it's just common sense'; 'it's always been that way'. But what is common sense? How does everyone know? And is this the way it has always been? The work of Alfred Schutz has been most influential in the exploration of the way meaning is built up in individual experience. I justify my appeal to both theoretical paradigms on the basis of my primary concern: to examine critically the taken-for-granted assumptions of staff, patients and others in relation to a broadly similar set of medical conditions, and to investigate these ideas as they become visible in social interaction over time.

Some of the analytical tools I have used need explanation here. A healthy person is transformed into a patient: a patient into a healthy person. But health itself is transformed, for the person, in the passage through a disease or injury syndrome. Transformation is the

> ...process of change and its completion whereby one context of meaning and action has its component elements and their particular ordering rearranged so as to constitute an altered, in effect transformed, context of meaning and action. A context comprises a matrix of elements and their relations, which together and in their interrelation constitute a particular framework of meaning...A transformation occurs when one context is changed into another. (Kapferer, 1979 ch.8)

This definition is consistent with my use of the term transformation in this book.

The words 'person' and 'patient' have established meanings in everyday usage. In this study I use these terms as labels to refer to the human actor at a certain stage in the transformation process. I certainly do not mean to imply that a patient is not a person. A person becomes a patient; a patient becomes a healthy person. His or her essential humanness is, of course, unaltered.

In this book, person and patient are analytical categories, marking the transformation of experience and meaning for the human actor.

A person may see him or herself, and be seen by others, as a patient simply because he or she is the subject of medical work. A visit to the dentist, a consultation at a family planning clinic, a smallpox vaccination or a bout of 'flu may lead a person to see him or herself as a patient, and allow others to designate him or her as such.

Such consultation to medically-oriented agencies, or episodes of transitory illhealth do not, however, involve a transformational process. In the passage of an individual through transitory illhealth the person moves from the context of health, through the context of disease, to the context of health again. But the processual movement from context to context does not involve a rearrangement of elements: one context is not changed into another. Rather, the context of health is de-emphasised as the person becomes a temporary patient, and this context is reinstated as the person understands his or her health to be restored.

If the disease process involves permanent destruction or alteration of skeletal or systemic function, a transformation of the meaning of health to the individual may occur. The former conception of health of the individual must be rearranged and reordered so as to constitute an altered context of meaning. A transformation of meaning occurs when one context is changed into another. Person and patient are labels marking the passage of the individual through the transformative processes.

The self—its construction, deconstruction and reconstruction—is an important theme of this study.

For G. H. Mead (1934), the self is the central mechanism with which the human being faces and deals with the world. The self arises from taking the 'attitude of the other' or the 'generalized other' (Mead, 1934:154). In mutual interrelationship, the self interacts with the other; the other interacts with the self. The point of intersection between the self and the other is the 'me'. The 'me' is the organised set of attitudes of others that one assumes (Mead, 1934:175). The self is constituted out of interaction between the 'I' and 'me' in a 'conversation of gestures' (Mead, 1934:167). Although the 'I' is personal, it is by no means independent of cultural expectations since it is built on the individual 'me' and since the individual always sees him or herself in relation to the community.

The 'reciprocity of perspectives' between self and other is

organised in relation to the cultural typifications relating to health in a particular context. Identification of a person as a patient establishes processes that subvert and reverse those processes that constructed the social self.

True rehabilitation, in contrast to the physical aspect of rehabilitation, depends on the full reconciliation of body and self. Until this union takes place, rehabilitation has not occurred. Through observing the experiences of paralysed people in this study, we can sense the feelings of distress that occur when the body and the self are estranged. Successful rehabilitation can only be achieved when the new body and the new self are united.

Rehabilitation now involves the shared knowledge and skills of many professional groups. Team work has been practised by traditional health workers—doctors, nurses, physiotherapists, social workers, occupational therapists—for some time. The introduction of anthropology, sociology and psychology into the curricula of health professionals is increasingly seen as an essential component of both undergraduate and post-graduate education. The rise of specialist rehabilitation workers in recent years has further emphasised the interdisciplinary nature of rehabilitation work and highlighted the necessity to attend to other issues beyond the physical restoration of function, which has achieved such excellence in spinal injuries and rehabilitation units throughout the world. Patients are becoming less willing to remain the passive recipients of professional work, a change that is welcomed by many health workers.

This study will, I hope, shed light on the patient's experience. It is unashamedly anthropological or sociological in nature. I hope that this will not deter the more pragmatic reader. The theory that I have used, like all theory, is only useful if it serves to illuminate or heighten our understanding of that which we usually take for granted. If it alienates the reader, or deters him or her from seriously considering the substance of this book, then it has failed in this aim. At this late stage of the twentieth century we can no longer afford to ignore the knowledge of other professional groups, or indeed, the insights of patients themselves. This book aims to integrate the special concerns of patients, social scientists and health professionals into an interrelated whole. No one group has a mandate to knowledge about body paralysis, or any other bodily disturbance, however temporary, with which men and women must reconcile themselves. We forget, sometimes, that as professional workers we have but one cause to serve—the needs of the patient. Let us listen to them.

2 The body and its activities

Throughout the ages the human body has been a rich and potent symbol in literature, art and the many creative works of men and women, both secular and sacred. The simplicity of the Greek kouros figures of the late seventh century and the later classical, yet no less beautiful, Roman sculptures bear witness to the admiration and attention that earlier cultures paid to the human body (Boardman, 1964:73). The devotion to the physical discipline of the body in warfare, sporting activities and the daily life of the ancient Greeks is further evidence of the central place of the body in these early civilisations.

The health and appearance of the human body, it seems, are no less important today than in former times. Our everyday lives are dominated by the existence of our bodies. Bodily activities—eating, washing, dressing and sleeping—are the major preoccupations of our lives. The body, its functions and malfunctions, is the focus of immense anxiety and concern.

The interior of the body is a context for anarchy. Our internal organs may turn against us—our cells may proliferate in mad disorder, our ducts block, our vessels rupture, or our glands cease to produce precious hormones. Our immune system, usually a paragon of vigilance, may destroy parts of the body of which it is itself a part. Articular cartilages may grind down, coronary and cerebral arteries occlude. Bits of body tissue may break off and do grave mischief in distant parts of the body. Valves may refuse to close, nerves cease to conduct, or more perversely, they may conduct bizarre and unpredictable messages.

Our well tended body may at any time betray our years of faithful love and care and grow some exotic virus within its enclosures. Seeds of disorder—parasites, fungi and bacteria—may be welcomed as guests within the organs and fluids, reservoirs and spaces of our body. Cells may take it upon themselves to grow—to expand, to push out other organs in their need for space—and when this space has been exhausted may spread into more and more of the body in their relentless, selfish quest for space and nourishment. Cachexia is the final capitulation of the body to these anarchic cells.

But this site of anarchy—the interior of my body—is inaccessible to me. How can I know if my cells and fluids, my nerves and cartilages are conspiring against me? Others must probe the depths of my body in order to reveal its innermost secrets. Doctors can search the reaches of the unknown, which I can never know, and choose whether or not to tell me what they find.

The exterior of the body is a much more public space, a calmer environment, more knowable, more controllable but also more controlled. The exterior of the body is the medium by which an individual represents him or herself in public. The self is constantly constituted in face to face interaction. Style and fashion are important tools of image management in a world that depends on outward signs of success. Survival in this competitive world depends on the selection of the most advantageous strategies for the presentation of the self.

Anxieties about the way we see ourselves and the way we wish others to see us concern us all from time to time. But seldom are these questions anything more than minor uncertainties in the normal course of our lives. If the image that confronts us from the bathroom mirror in the morning is displeasing, the modern fashion and cosmetics industries have provided us with a myriad of tools with which we can swiftly effect changes in our appearance to make it conform to our idea of how we wish others to see us. The brush, the comb, hair spray and makeup of all kinds will emphasise those parts that are valued and hide those likely to meet with less approval.

The range of variables in the garments with which we choose to clothe ourselves is enormous and complex. Not only do such garments conceal or reveal aspects of our body to others, but by our choice and manipulation of these details we have the power to effect considerable control over the way we appear to others. High heels, flat heels, boots or bare feet represent simple ways of altering not only our height but also our impression on others.

I am not suggesting that everyone has equal opportunity to construct their social appearance through the use of these commercial devices. One has only to catch a glimpse of the Royal Enclosure at Ascot, opening night at the opera, or the Melbourne Cup on television to realise that such instruments are strongly linked to class. Nevertheless, many of the tools of appearance manipulation are widely available, and can be used to satisfy any temporary discrepancy in the way we see ourselves and the way we would like others to see us. Such discrepancies can normally be redressed without disrupting the semblance of consistency for which most of us strive.

Clothing may well not be enough. The art of the beautician, hairdresser, dentist, aerobics instructor, manicurist and dietician may be needed to create the bodily showcase of the successful self. Plastic reconstructive surgery is a more radical, but quite common recourse of reconciliation of external body appearance and self-image. Such body manipulations are no idiosyncratic personal whim—these activities are structurally motivated decisions which people make in order to enhance their opportunities at work and at play—to improve their chances in society. The self is a visible self; the body is draped, decorated, moulded, shaped and styled or even neglected in order to represent clearly and overtly the status of the self.

The body has also been a source of perennial sociological concern. Although the spectre of biological reductionism has discouraged an interest in the body by many sociologists, other social analysts see the body as central to sociology.

Within a society there is usually widespread agreement about what men and women should be like, about what physical states can be described as normal. There is a shared understanding of what in that society constitutes a healthy, a beautiful or an erotic body. Marcel Mauss in his 'Techniques of the human body' (1936) extended this Durkheimian view of society to explore how social meaning is grafted onto the physical medium of the human body. Through the processes of training and education the human body is transformed into a social artifact. 'In every society, everyone knows and has to know and learn what he has to do in all conditions' (Mauss, 1936:85). Following in the Durkheimian tradition Mary Douglas extends this thesis further. 'The social body constrains the way the physical body is perceived' (Douglas, 1970:93). Our perception of the experiences of our own body is socially determined. The experience of the functioning of our body is not universally the same: the experience varies in different social contexts and at different historical times. Yet within a social context and at a particular historical time there is widespread communal understanding about the attributes, functioning and experiences of the human body.

The sociologists of the Durkheimian school examined people's understandings of the human body in order to understand people's other, social body—society (Douglas, 1970:93–112).

14 Bodily alterations

This was their focus of inquiry. If the human body is always treated as an image of society then much can be learned about a society by determining people's attitudes to their bodies.

My primary focus in this book is the other side of this equation, the human body—the research tool the Durkheimians used to investigate their primary concern, society itself. Our private self is housed within a public body. Society influences our attitudes towards our own bodies and those of others. Training and education transform our bodies into socially recognisable objects. The physiological functioning of our body is experienced differently in different social contexts. The human body is thoroughly embedded within the social body.

We have bodies, but we are bodies. Our embodiment is essential for our social being. A person experiences him or herself as an entity not identical with the body, but one that has a body at his or her disposal (Berger and Luckman, 1967:68). The inextricable relationship between body as being and body as resource contributes to the interest invested in the human body, and the power of the body as a metaphor for different societies throughout the ages.

I can touch, feel, smell and see my body, but I need my body in order carry out these acts of touching, feeling, smelling and seeing. I possess my body in a much more thorough and immediate sense than I could ever possess other objects. Yet although I possess my body in this thoroughgoing sense, the very intimacy of possession is the source of my destruction, since the death of my body is also my death. Disease that involves loss of bodily function or control challenges the intimacy of the relationship between body as being and body as resource, and can constitute a most profound form of human alienation (Turner, 1984:233), as this study will explore.

I develop an awareness of my body by my experience of living in my body and by means of my various senses, which inform me about my own body. But the body in which I live is visible to others, it is the object of social attention. I learn about my body from the impressions I see my body make on other people. These interactions with others provide critical visual data for my self-knowledge.

An image in the mirror adds another dimension of knowledge about myself. It offers a perspective that approximates, but never exactly represents, my corporeal self-image. The image in the mirror offers the first intimation of alienation from my own inner awareness. I am no longer what I feel myself to be. On seeing the image I leave the reality of the lived me, and come to refer myself to the ideal, fictitious or imaginary me, which has been suggested by this first alter-image in the mirror. I am, in a sense, torn from myself (Merleau-Ponty, 1964:136–7). The image in the mirror foreshadows more serious alienation—my alienation from others. Others will have an exterior image of me, comparable to the image in the mirror, but unlike the inanimate mirror, others are capable of reacting to me on the basis of this image of me that they see. The reactions of others can complete an image of me that I can only partially experience: '...saying that I have a body is thus a way of saying that I can be seen as an object and that I try to be seen as a subject, that another can be my master or my slave...' (Merleau-Ponty, 1962:167).

More recently, Turner (1984), influenced by the work of French philosopher Michel Foucault, has refocussed sociological interest in the centrality of the body. For Turner the problem of social order can be restated as a problem of government of the body—the regimen or government of a given society is seen in parallel with the regimen or government of the body. Social order depends on the resolution of the perpetual tension between desire and control, between anarchy and civilisation, between the body and social regulation.

The nature–culture dichotomy, a prevailing theme in sociology, is critical to this argument. By virtue of their bodies, human beings are a part of nature; because they also have minds they are simultaneously part of culture. Culture modifies and reorders nature. A 'natural' body expression in one society may have a totally different meaning in another. Anthropological data provides us with a wealth of examples of culturally specific behaviours, gestures and body expressions. Japanese people spit in public, but do not blow their noses (Turner, 1984:204). Looking a person squarely in the eye is seen as a sign of integrity in Western society, but as a mark of serious disrespect in some parts of the world.

The tension between these two domains—nature and culture—is the source of much social concern. Civilised life is achieved by controlling and constraining nature, a victory that is always tentative, always susceptible to overthrow. The potential anarchy of striving for biological satisfaction must be subordinated by a variety of institutional controls (Turner, 1984:61). The body needs food, drink and sleep. The nature, content and

16 Bodily alterations

timing of eating, drinking and sleeping, however, are heavily socially regulated. Similarly, the body of the individual is constrained and regulated in the interests of the wider society. Every society develops complex regulations prescribing the variabilities of human sexuality. Incest taboos and rules concerning abortion, infanticide, illegitimacy and homosexuality are some of the measures by which culture constrains nature for the good of society. Social order depends on the subordination of physical desires to the rationality of the mind through such agencies as the family, the church and the state (Foucault, 1981).

Over time, the nature–culture dichotomy has also provided powerful explanations for the social subordination of women. Because of woman's monopoly on reproduction she is clearly associated with nature. 'Natural' attributes—maternal instincts and emotions—derive from her relationship with her body and with nature. Man's distance from the pragmatics of reproduction aligns him, de facto, with culture. This alliance provides him with controlled reason, reliability, rationality—attributes essential to life in the 'real' world, the public domain—in contrast to the private domestic world of child bearing and caring, the world of women.

Certainly biological differences do exist between men and women, but gender identity is further emphasised by socialisation into specific gender roles and attitudes. Being masculine means, quite literally, to embody force and competence. Force and competence are translations into the language of the body of social relations that define men as holders of power, women as subordinate. Through the constant exercising undertaken by boys and the social constraints that inhibit girls from similar activities these statements become embedded in the body, not just in mental body images, but in the very feel and texture of the body, its attitudes, its muscular tensions, its surfaces (Connell, 1983:38).

Similarly, the processes of maturation and degeneration of the body are functions of nature. However, the categories of infant, child, adolescent and old person are cultural products strongly influenced by structural forces; they constitute meaningful stages of life in a world of cultural beliefs, symbols and practices.

The frailty, vulnerability and inevitable demise of the human body are continual themes in religion. A perilous equilibrium exists between nature and culture, between biology and society, between natural depravity and divine purity. The body is weak, and must be continually on guard against the sins of the flesh.

Despite God's injunction to care for the sick, aged and infirm, the duty to be healthy by mastery of the flesh became an important outward sign of inward spiritual virtue. A healthy body is implicit in the concept of salvation. The most powerful symbol of the profane world is the disordered human body. The body is dangerous. Bodily secretions, particularly semen and menstrual blood, have to be shielded by ritual and taboo to protect the social order. Yet at the same time, the body is sacred. The sacrifice of Christ's body, a sacrifice for our salvation, is symbolised by wine and bread. The body and blood are redistributed at the Holy Eucharist.

Eating is another basic activity in which the body and society are held in an uneasy tension between desire and control. Through a myriad of cultural categories and prescriptions we learn what constitutes appropriate food in a particular society, how it should be prepared, how much should be consumed and how we should eat it. Jewish dietary laws may surprise the outsider unfamiliar with their logic, yet we seldom ponder the origin of many of our own dietary categories and eating behaviours. Complex forms of etiquette govern not only how we should manipulate spoons, forks and knives, but also who should sit by one's right hand and in which direction a man should pass the port.

Both the eating and sharing of food are powerful media of social relations. Anniversaries, celebrations and social events involve food sharing, particular foods become associated with particular commemorations. To fail to offer at least a drink to a visitor to your house may be seen as an act of serious social impropriety. Taking a friend out to dinner, or bringing an intended partner to eat with the family are events of great significance in personal relationships. The privileges that evolve from sharing food at a business lunch or at a private dinner party, though difficult to quantify, are not hard to imagine.

Feeding a child is a fundamental activity of parental care and support. An infant depends entirely on its parents for nutritional sustenance. A baby cries because it is hungry, but the way a parent chooses to assuage the baby's hunger is heavily influenced by the culture in which the parent lives. Whether the baby is offered a breast or a bottle, whether it will be fed on demand or must wait four hours for the next feed, whether it will be solid foods at three months or not until the child has cut the first tooth are elements of culture to which the parent is responding. It will not be long before the child learns that there is no point in crying for food now because its parents have clearly decided to feed on a four-hourly schedule. The baby's digestive system learns to need food at four-hourly intervals. In a sense, society has invaded the child's body and rearranged the function of its anatomy to conform to a particular set of social ideas.

Toilet training and sleep training are obvious examples of similar social subordination of physiological function. Parental authority in subsequent areas of life can be seen to develop out of these dependency relations.

As we grow up we gain control over our feeding patterns—we can choose what, when, how and with whom to eat. But although these choices constitute significant personal autonomy, they in fact represent a choice between a relatively small range of options provided by the culture in which we live. Refusing to eat is a powerful act of social rebellion. By means of hunger strikes and anorexia nervosa the body asserts its supremacy over society in a stand that can easily become a pyrrhic victory. Similarly, the obese body has come to signify a body out of control, and the eating disorder bulimia represents a personal expression of the tension between desire and the social criteria of appropriate body size and shape, especially for women.

Growing up is a process of social transformation. The child takes in the world through bodily experiences. One by one a baby's body movements are captured by social forces. The baby's eyes learn to focus, its arms to reach out toward some object of desire, and its smile loses its randomness and directs its effect towards significant others. Gradually the involuntary gestures and movements, the body flexures and inertias of the newborn baby are replaced by the vitality and purposeful activity of the maturing person. A person demonstrates maturity by intentional body movement. The physical development of the body constrains the rate of identity formation, though even this is socially influenced in terms of the amount of freedom given to the child.

Sitting, standing and walking are important milestones in a child's development towards adulthood. The adult posture is upright—the erect body is a product of skeletal and muscular action. But the upright posture is heavily enmeshed in moral postures (Sacks, 1986:98). Standing up for oneself, being upright and standing tall are metaphors for a person's social status. Similarly, the movement of the upright body—walking—is a powerful metaphor for social independence. Walking symbolises the movement away from the dependencies of childhood towards the independence of adult status. A grown child walks away from his or her parents, a mature person walks away from those upon whom he or she depended.

Traditionally, human societies have defined the boundary between nature and culture by a variety of ritual arrangements. Rituals of inclusion such as baptism, circumcision and scarification transform the natural body into a social entity and invite access to a whole range of rights and statuses that are the privilege of membership of that particular society. The actions of washing, burning and cutting transform the natural body, and provide evidence to others of the inclusion of the person into the body of society.

Similarly, the transfer of the body out of culture, back to nature at the end of social life, is associated with rituals of exclusion. Through burial and cremation ceremonies a person's social being is deconstructed in a way that suggests that he or she is becoming more natural—that he or she is returning, from 'dust to dust', from 'ashes to ashes'. Death brings to an end the complex roles and relationships of social life. Technical advances in modern medicine have blurred the division between life and death, but clinical death remains quite distinct from social death, which may occur much earlier. This distinction raises profound ethical dilemmas, dilemmas that society must address in the near future.

What we know depends on language. What exists for us is dependent on language and the explicatory resources made available to us by a particular linguistic system. Our experience of our body can only be known to us by means of the classification systems devised by our culture. Bodies are part of nature: the body is essentially biological. But explanations based on biology are never sufficient explanation of human behaviour or action. The body is also a social construction; it is heavily influenced by social forces in a social context. Biology, physiology, anatomy are in themselves part of culture, not nature. They are the classificatory systems devised by society to organise and systematise human experience. Our understanding, our knowledge of the body is not an innate understanding of a natural organism, but is knowledge mediated through the social auspices of biology, physiology and anatomy.

Sexuality is experienced not as a stirring of interior physiology, but as a learned feature of sexual ideology in a particular social context at a particular historical time. Similarly hunger, though undoubtedly physiological at base, is embedded in a cultural superstructure of enormous complexity. Culture, though, is never a neutral vehicle. Language, and the classificatory systems that evolve from language, reflect structural interests in society. Some groups in society have more power, and thereby have greater potential to assert that their definitions of reality are seen as the reality.

How then do we come to know ourselves, how do others know us, and how do we learn our place in the world?

Socialisation is the process by which we acquire our social characteristics and by which we learn the ways of thought and behaviour considered appropriate in our society. Socialisation continues throughout life; this learning process ends only when social life itself ends—with death.

The family is a crucial influence in the development of attitudes and behaviours in the growing child. The power of this primary socialisation is formidable—formidable because it is informal, unaccounted for, and because the participants in the process are most often united by bonds of proximity, genetics and familial love. Through observation and experience of daily life in the family, a child learns about its body, the meaning of different anatomical parts and the acceptable way of controlling its functions.

At school a child learns not only traditional subjects, but also a whole range of codes and practices regulating behaviour. In addition to learning mathematics and physics, the student also learns how to relate to the teacher, how to present him or herself when asking for an extension of time for an assignment, how to look interested in what is being said. A student who learns the value of these visible modes of bodily expression, this 'hidden curriculum', is likely to fare much better in the education system than a student who does not understand their social power.

So we learn very early in our formal education what we can do with our body to elicit approval and what we should do to avoid disapproval. We acquire valuable social skills about how to respond to those in authority. Our bodies learn how to display to others a visual representation of a state of mind. Through habit the outward representation mostly conforms to the inner attitude, but not always. We learn how to manage the face and body in order to look a certain way, so that they will express socially valued meanings that enhance our ability to live with others in groups. Such influential aspects of social interaction are learned informally and unintentionally, as products of the powerful yet unaccounted learning that takes place in the family, and later in the peer group and classroom.

Patterns of behaviour and bodily expression knit together to form a consistent whole. Certain attributes and modes of presentation come to represent categories of people within society. Although speaking and accent are probably the most obvious interactional symbols of class, many more subtle activities such as facial expressions and body gestures indicate class difference no less directly. Learned displays of gender—girlish behaviour, boyish behaviour—are laid down firmly within the family and constantly elaborated upon by peers, the media, teachers and others thoughout life. Age, like gender, has biological substance, but that substance in it self is not sufficient to explain the complex expressional forms that different age groups engender. Acting out age—taking on the dominant social expressions and presentations of the body considered to be appropriate to that age—is seen by many people to be more detrimental to ageing people than the actual biological degeneration that may occur.

Although definite consistencies in bodily expression exist between categories of people within society, as individuals we respond to others by trying to modify our behaviour in order to please, shock, embarrass, placate, annoy or merely to satisfy the other person. We vary our behaviour to suit the particular person with whom we are relating, and also to substantiate in a more general sense our legitimate membership of the broad social category to which we belong, or to which we aspire. By their hair style and colour, their dress and bodily demeanor, punk rockers are stating to others their disrespect for dominant social categories, but also their unity with other people who feel the same. Twin sets and tweed skirts, business suits and ties are common but powerful symbols of conformity to the status quo.

More formal manipulation of bodily expression occurs when a person intentionally takes on the dress, styles, gestures, postures and expressions of a group he or she wishes to join. A young woman from a working-class background may deliberately reject the patterns of dress, behaviour and leisure activities of her childhood in order to attract a more economically comfortable middle-class partner. Many women have chosen to renounce the superficial trappings of femininity, those qualities seen as inherently feminine before the women's movement, and have lost none of their womanliness for it.

Immense industries survive and prosper on the manipulation

of the outward and visible symbols of age. Such activities range from the enormous commerce devoted to the presentation of baby as a most significant domestic product, to the hugely profitable adolescent market in clothes, jewellery, make-up and other impedimenta whereby a teenager may express him or herself as a properly socialised, fully legitimate member of this social group.

Capitalism, geared to production, reproduction and the construction of needs and desires finds the older person hard to place in its productive system. By marginalising old people from the mainstream of its productive forces, capitalism has in turn created a profound fear of age, which serves as a profitable force for the very economic system that created it. Fear of ageing in a society that deals so badly with ageing people has spawned huge capitalist enterprises that make products to manipulate the outward signs of an ageing body. Dress, body ornaments, and of course the cosmetic industry hold out the promise, if not of eternal youth, then at least a few more years of heavenly grace.

Social existence is precarious. Although the process of internalisation explains why most social rules are obeyed most of the time, knowledge of the rules and standards of a group does not always ensure conformity. Legal sanctions such as fines, detentions, banishments and gaol underwrite the socialisation process. Informal sanctions, however, may be much more powerful reinforcements to those rules we learned in childhood. Conformity in our society most often brings its own reward. Most people desire, and actively seek, the approval of others. For this reason gossip, ostracism, satire and ridicule are formidable sanctions against non-conforming behaviour. These tools of social control are well documented by anthropologists in small communities, but I defy the reader to deny the continuing power of such mechanisms in our complex industrial society.

Yet despite these powerful social rules and sanctions, the individual has a mind capable of understanding and interpreting what other people mean by their social actions. Rather than a simple process of internalisation of rules, social behaviour is learned and negotiated in a more interactive manner, a manner which by its nature incorporates change and diversity (Bilton et al., 1981:25). Creative and innovative action evolves from such interactions. New definitions of the situation may arise, new interpretations of behaviour become possible in this perspective that underlies this study.

A cautionary note should be introduced here lest we overestimate the possibilities for individual intellect and action. We do have the potential to be creative, but only within the limitations of our socially created selves. Our selves are created in interaction with others in a social context. The self is thus constrained by the dimensions of the context from which it arises, and by forces of socialisation influencing other individuals with whom we interact. The values and attitudes perpetuated through the socialising agencies are not neutral messages. Socialisation is predicated on the dominant views of certain groups in society who have the power to make their definition of reality *the* reality. Class socialisation and gender socialisation thus act to bind the less priviledged members of society to the beliefs and ideas that legitimate the status quo. The world view, beliefs, attitudes and values of the dominant class become the beliefs, attitudes and values of all members of society. These views become the structures of the individual conscience, the vantage point from which the individual evaluates aspects of society. Thus choice can never be free of the constraints inherent in our social being. Individual decisions and actions are prescribed by such structural considerations.

Central to this study is the critical interrelationship between body, mind and social context. The interdependancy is brought into critical relief when the usual balance between these three components is disturbed. Morbidity of the body enables us to witness a breakdown in the usual conceptual and social processes that sustain the status quo. Permanent body paralysis provides a dramatic and highly visible research tool to observe the essentiality of the mind–body–society triumvirate. The taken for granted nature of this relationship is revealed in dramatic form when the normal functioning of one component of the triumvirate can no longer be assumed.

The human body is thoroughly embedded within the social world. Realisation that social norms are not concrete categories but are socially constructed and continually changing may allow the person with a disability at least a small degree of liberation from their oppressive presence.

3 Health and illhealth

What is health? How do we know that we are healthy? How do we feel when we are well? Words like 'great', 'fine', or even 'terrific!' seem quite inadequate to convey the reality of good health—the unthinking confidence that our limbs will move and that our organs will continue to function, the careless assumptions we hold about the vitality of our bodies.

An idea of health is something everyone has. Yet although 'everyone knows' what health is for themselves, precise definition of this attribute seems impossible. The World Health Organisation (WHO) defines health as '...a state of complete physical, mental and social wellbeing, and not merely the absence of disease and infirmity'. Modern medicine uses highly sophisticated tests and investigations to reach a verdict of good health. But most people do not use scientific criteria to evaluate their own health, and the WHO definition is meaningless to the majority of the world's population.

Ambiguity exists about the meaning of the term because there is no set of features common to all healthy people. Health is a social construction. What we call health results from the interaction between an individual and his or her social context. Health cannot be ascribed to people by official agencies. People understand themselves to be healthy, or understand their health to be deficient. No external designation of health will have any meaning unless it is perceived to be so by the people concerned. What is experienced as health represents a complex of intimate and cultural understandings in a particular social context, not a fixed set of physiological and biochemical facts.

The ideas of health which people hold are a product of the wider structural forces operating in the social context in which they arise. Each individual has a part in constructing his or her world, but institutional forms of social organisation, social groups, and systems of status and prestige precede the existence of each individual. Because these structures 'have always been there', they take on the nature of taken for granted objectivities (Berger and Luckman, 1967:77). These structures prescribe the manner in which an individual comprehends his or her world. But such comprehension is never neutral. Knowledge is socially differentiated in terms of the structural differentiation of society (Wagner, 1970:ch.11).

Within a social context knowledge is sorted into various zones of relevance (Wagner, 1970:111). In addition, the multitudes of phemonena in the world are ordered into a limited number of classes or groups. This grouping constitutes typification. Through this socially approved system of typifications and relevances (Wagner, 1970:120), the individual relates his or her intimate, personal experiences to the broader spheres of pre-established cultural interpretations, and orients him or herself to the social world.

Cultural yardsticks are used to measure and interpret physical well being. People use cultural constructions to evaluate and interpret, to give meaning to their self-conceptions of health. Different cultural understanding influence the way an individual perceives, interprets and responds to symptoms. Certain ideas predominate among members of particular subgroups within a society. Since there is no inherent physiological difference between the members of different social classes or ethnic groups, variations in health and illness ideas, and in the type of social action likely to evolve, are related to these typifications (Zola, 1973:680).

Childbirth, for example, is experienced differently in our society and Papua New Guinea. Western woman feels more pain in childbirth. But this does not mean that Western women are imagining their pain nor that Papua New Guinean women are especially stoic. It is part of Western cultural knowledge that childbirth is temporarily disabling and can endanger the life of the mother and child. There is no simple relationship between the objectively assessable severity of a symptom and the individual's experience of pain and discomfort. Recognition of a symptom as a problem, and the action considered appropriate to deal with it, are components of cultural knowledge. But the woman's previous experiences, her assessment of the effectiveness of a certain action and the severity of the symptom itself, are also important components of the way symptoms are experienced.

The cultural constructions and typifications through which

people communicate and interpret their experience of health are important because they also influence people's ideas about disease. What motivates an individual to enter into remedial action? When, why and how does the individual see his or her health as a problem? Which features of a person's conception of health are singled out at a particular time as important, and which components are suppressed? What benefits does an individual hope to achieve by a particular action? And when does he or she feel health to be restored?

An individual develops a construction of him or herself as a healthy person in terms of a complex interplay between bodily experiences, cultural constructions and typifications, and the everyday understandings of others. This social construction is by no means static, but is an ongoing, continually modified process.

Current popular culture places great value on individual health and physical fitness. An enormous commercial industry provides the means for people to appear healthy. 'Good health', or a social construction of good health, is not only chic, but clearly demonstrates to others that the individual is a responsible citizen. Cults of male physicality—football, surfing, body building and the martial arts—provide the means for men to create the appearance of healthy masculinity, which is synonymous with the social power structure of patriarchy (Connell, 1983:38). Similarly, the physical culture movement in early twentieth-century England provided the vehicle for the creation of a modern representation of women's bodies (Matthews, 1987).

Contemporary goals are health, success and self-fulfillment. 'Finding yourself' is an urgent priority; one does this through a single-minded and energetic devotion to one's own body (Lynch, 1987:129). The intensely individualistic nature of endeavours to reach this goal—activities such as aerobics, rigorous weight reduction programmes, reconstructive surgery—suggest the development of an identity that is isolated from socio-cultural influences, a disembodiment—a denial of a person's past and lived experience (Lynch, 1987:139).

Yet the appearance of good health has not always been desirable. Nineteenth-century social acceptability was guaranteed by an antithetical image. The romanticising of tuberculosis gave social merit to those people who appeared sick. It was fashionable to be pale and drained. The tubercular look had to be considered attractive once it came to be considered a mark of distinction and breeding (Sontag, 1979:57). The dreadful reality of tuberculosis was distorted and denied in order to express romantic attitudes about the self.

My task of detaching the taken for granted notions of health and illhealth from their status as established, objectivated realities has established the socially-constructed nature of such categories, the continually changing manner of their construction, and their differential perception at any one time by groups and individuals with society.

Health and illhealth have no reality in their own right. They cannot be recognised in unambiguous terms. They have no substance, no independent being apart from meanings that emerge through individual experience and social factors in relation to others in a particular social context. Grand ideas about what health is must be suspended. Exploration of the manner in which health is defined, who does the defining, what health means to people, and how ideas of health are used in social action is a much more critical activity. To establish the multidimensional, multivalent and processual nature of health is an essential preliminary to an exploration of people's understandings of themselves as not healthy, and their subsequent understandings of their renewed health after the bodily alterations that are the subject of this book.

What, then, is illhealth? Health, it seems, is typified as a taken for granted state of normalcy. Illhealth, then, implies a divergence from normal, an undesirable state of disruption.

Naturalistic theories of illhealth have existed in many societies for a very long time. and are based on the premise that good health depends on a balance between people and nature, a precarious equilibrium that requires constant vigilance. The three major naturalistic explanatory frameworks are humoral pathology, Ayurvedic medicine and traditional Chinese medicine (Morgan, Calnan and Manning, 1985:ch.1). For our purposes the elaborate humoral theory can be reduced to four essential components—elements, qualities, humours and temperaments. In this theory health is the result of a fine balance between the four elements: earth, air, fire and water; the four qualities of matter: cold, hot, wet and dry; the four body fluids or humours: blood, black bile, yellow bile and phlegm; and the four temperaments associated with these humours: sanguine, melancholic, choleric and phlegmatic. This balance can be upset by a disturbance of any of the component elements, by natural forces as well as by strong emotions. Illness in men and women results from this disequilibrium, this lack of harmony between natural and bodily elements. Treatments arising from this explanatory system involve removal of some of the incriminating fluid or humour from the body in order to restore the balance between the humours. Emetics, purges and blood letting were common strategies for restoring bodily order. Such ideas persisted in Europe throughout the middle ages and into the seventeenth century.

Ayurvedic medicine shows many similarities with humoral pathology. Good health in this explanatory frame work results from a satisfactory balance between three doshas—phlegm, bile and flatulence. Traditional Chinese medicine also highlights the importance of equilibrium between different elements, specifically, yin and yang (Morgan, Calnan and Manning, 1985:ch.1).

It is not hard to discern remnants of these influential naturalistic theories of health and illhealth in many contemporary 'alternative' health practices. Certainly, in positing a critical relationship between environment, body and emotions such frameworks come much closer to foreshadowing a social perspective of health and illness than many of the subsequent theories that became the precursors of modern medicine.

Health, then, is normal. Health is life in balance with nature. Health is order. Illhealth is thus abnormal, a body out of balance with nature, in disarray and dirorder. Health is the resolution of the tension between bodily control and social control: it results from the regulation of the anarchy of the body by the civilising forces of society. Hygiene, exercise, diet, sleep regulation and sexual continence are socially developed practices of body regulation designed to ensure a healthy, normal, well ordered body, a body that will not by its difference threaten the status quo. This is not to imply that all healthy people are social conformists, but in our contemporary context those people who seek to help themselves by engaging in these clearly defined practices will gain social approval for their actions and sympathy should they become ill. Clearly such practices are as much political as they are functional. The regulation of the body is conducive to social order.

Illness and disease can be seen as a result of the body's inability or refusal to conform to society's prescriptions. If health is normalcy, illhealth is deviancy—the unhealthy person is a deviant. Social order can be directly related to the issue of regulation of the body. Social order depends on the resolution of the perpetual tension between desire and discipline, between anarchy and order, between the body and society (Turner,

1984). Health, in similar terms, depends on the resolution of the same tensions. Illness indicates that the equilibrium between these principles has been violated. Disease is the most salient metaphor of structural crisis (Turner, 1984:114). Illness is dangerous. Illness not only causes a breakdown in the usual roles and obligations generated by social life, but, more importantly, illness challenges the hegemony of the status quo—it demonstrates that the normative order of society is not immutable. A disordered body disrupts the social order. By its existence a disordered body may point to new realities.

The meaning of certain illnesses reflect anxieties about acceptable and unacceptable social behaviour from the perspective of the dominant social group. Anorexia nervosa is a clear example of the conflicting demands of female gender in contemporary society (Turner, 1984:112), while sexually-transmitted diseases of all kinds, but most dramatically AIDS, have provoked extreme anxiety about acceptable sexual behaviour.

Health, 'normal health', is thus inextricable from society and from the power relations in society. The manner in which we define our bodies, and subsequently the way we come to see our body as unhealthy is directly influenced by society. The body states that come to be seen as normal are those states that conform to the ideas of a dominant group in society. A body out of order indicates that society is out of order. If such a deviation cannot be managed, then the unhealthy body will have to be marginalised—pushed to the periphery of society, not accounted for, out of sight—lest it should distract others from devotion to the dominant ideology, which is health and normalcy.

In the past, and indeed in many non-industrial societies today, a shaman or witchdoctor mediated the restoration of balance between the body and nature. Today in our society medicine mediates. Medicine is a formidable agency of social order. Medicine restores the dangerous, disordered, unhealthy body to health. Medicine neutralises the major source of deviance in society—illness (Richman, 1987:ch.3). The management of mental illnesses, reproduction and sexually-transmitted diseases in particular demonstrates medicine's critical role in balancing society's tensions. A doctor mediates between desire and control, between anarchy and order, and in so doing reaffirms the status quo.

Turner (1984:211). claims that medicine has replaced religion as the social guardian of morality. Modern medicine implies that a certain asceticism is the main defence against sexually-transmitted disease, heart disease, stress and cancer (Turner,

1984:214). The medicalisation of the body, the appropriation of the body and its activities by medicine, especially in such critical domains as sexuality, reproduction, eating, drinking, sleeping and 'correct' thinking, has provided a formidable moral framework for life, maybe more powerful than religion in the past since it posits a more immediate horror than hell—disease in the here and now.

The relationship between health and morality, the notion that improper life styles are the cause of personal illness, has enjoyed a long vogue. The dire warnings about the consequences of masturbation and other sexual practices in Victorian times were indications of the moral anxieties of this era. Modern medicine, however, has not abandoned the shackles of such moral imperatives. Despite its claims to scientific objectivity, the contribution of 'a healthy lifestyle' to physical well being is omnipresent. Sexually-transmitted diseases such as herpes, gonorrhoea, cervical cancer and AIDS can be avoided if the individual controls his or her sexual passions, practices only certain kinds of sexual activity, is monogamous or, even better, celibate. Many other illnesses and disease states carry similar medico-moral underpinnings, but never so clearly as those connected with sexuality— clearly a recurrent anxiety in our era, which has had to publicly address such issues as homosexuality, contraceptive freedom and equality of women.

Disease is seen as retribution for an unhealthy life, the moral deviant becomes sick through his or her own behaviour, either by carelessness or design. We can choose to be well, or we can choose to be sick. Disease can be controlled by social hygiene and by our rigorous attention to our bodily habits in regard to exercise, ingestion, sleep and sexuality. Carelessness or neglect of such personal body routines will incur social approbation, such anti-social behaviour will be stigmatised.

The idea that germs and viruses are indiscriminate in their search for a host is powerful reinforcement for compliance in practices of body regulation. The individual's only defence against these random infective agents is to keep his or her body in good order. This idea obscures the fact that some people in society are much more likely to become sick than others. Class, gender, age and ethnicity are powerful social variables influencing our susceptibility to illhealth, and also affecting our likelihood of getting well. As Mitchell says (1984), illness is not a natural disaster, but is highly socially organised. The open drains, crowded living conditions, polluted water and harsh employment practices that made up the disease medium of the nineteenth century have gone, but only to be replaced by similar disease-producing environments in this century. Now, as at the end of the nineteenth century, our health is intimately linked with the conditions of our lives, with the socio-economic organisation of society.

'Lifestyle' has become the primary target of illness preventative activity. Such a focus does not, alas, refer to the broad sense of the word; the manner in which a person lives his or her life in conjunction with others in a society at a particular time. Rather, this usage reflects a much more restricted meaning of the term lifestyle, a highly individualistic and insular connotation, and thus represents a mere detached fragment of the real issue of illness in society.

Lifestyle strategies are based on the premise that people are their own worst enemies. By their careless disrespect for the basic techniques of body regulation, people inflict illhealth and disease upon themselves. Not surprisingly, 'bad' lifestyle practices correlate with working-class people, 'good' practices with the middle class, or with aspirants to that class. 'Sensible people' take the advice doctors give them, they have the intelligence to know what is good for them and the self-control to resist health damaging practices. They give up smoking, take up jogging and eat low-cholesterol foods. Others live from day to day, they smoke, drink and hang about. They are promiscuous, not interested in contraception, and they ignore the advice of health professionals (Mitchell, 1984:97). Abundant evidence proves that people with the least power in society also suffer the worst health. In times of rapidly escalating medical costs the perceived illness-producing behaviour of such people is an obvious target for modificatory activities.

Exercise, diet, sobriety, sexual continence and stress reduction are some of the measures an individual may employ to defend his or her body against illness. Of course these activities have some undeniable benefits, but to suggest that these measures will alleviate illness is to operate within an extremely simplistic perspective of health and illhealth. More importantly, it deflects attention away from the structural determinants of illhealth and, should the individual become ill, it implies that the victim is to blame for his or her disease or disability.

Health and illhealth result from a complexity of social, political, economic, ecological and gender variables as well as a range of biographical, physical and psychological factors within a social context at a particular historical time. To suggest that an activity like exercise can play anything more than a minor role in the prevention of disease denies the social nature of disease, and reduces both health and illhealth to ridiculously simplistic concepts. Such suggestions may of course offer a semblance of control over a person's life, but the cost of such comfort may be the diversion of attention away from the real sources of disease. It lets polluters, bad road designers, pharmaceutical manufacturers, urban planners and many other potential illness-producing agents off the hook. Such practices continue unabated, while people who become ill are burdened with guilt because they believe that they have caused their disease by failing to defend their bodies in a satisfactory manner. Their guilt is not only self-imposed: others will also blame them for their condition, and before long insurance companies and similar agencies will reinforce this guilt by refusing to do business with people who can be seen to be responsible for their own conditions.

The goal to which practitioners of the 'lifestyle' paradigm of health promotion aspire is epitomised in a visual image of a healthy body. The success of such programmes is evaluated by indices of the appearance of health. Commercial tools, especially the media, set the criteria for health by which we all are judged. Such commercial representations of health—a healthy look—may have very little to do with actual health, yet are extremely influential on peoples perceptions of themselves and others. It is not surprising that health promotion teams often include a person familiar with advertising. Ironically, the images used to promote health are often identical with the images used to promote cigarettes, alcohol and other health-denying products.

Health promotion and illness prevention are extremely conservative endeavours. By focussing on the individual, such agencies obscure the activities of governments and other structural agencies that beg scrutiny. Such an isolationist perspective of a 'vacuum packed' individual denies that individuals are human—that they act and interact in complex networks and develop sophisticated understandings of events in a world filled with other people.

The liaison between psychology and medicine is largely responsible for the individualistic strategies undertaken by health promotion and illness prevention programmes. Such practices, landlocked as they are by the intellectual bases of these disciplines, ignore the effects of social structure and history on health, illness and disability. As such they can never produce change, there is no way out of their narrow parameters. By continuing to focus on the individual as the source of his or her health and illhealth, such perspectives become entrenched in the inevitabilities of their own theoretical bases, and obscure the wider parameters of health and illhealth from view. They deny the inextricable relationship between mind, body and society.

The behavioural modification strategies most often used in health promotion programmes imply that the key to salvation of the body lies in individual behaviour. Men and women have bodies, but such strategies deny the obvious fact that men and women's bodies exist in an environment—in an environment of winds and storms, of currents and sunshine—an environment of pollens and spores. Even though these elements can be seen as 'natural', very little that happens in nature is in fact natural. Floods generally happen because men or women have altered water courses, fires usually occur because we inadvertently or wilfully light them—they spread because we have changed the ecology to suit our needs. More critically, men and women live in a social environment—a world of class, of politics and economics—hardly a neutral environment. Some people in society clearly have more power, and thus more opportunities than others. Access to resources affects peoples' access to power, which provides access to many other opportunities in society— most notably, the opportunity to maintain health. An individual is thoroughly embedded in his or her social world. To suggest that a minute aspect of behavioural modification is likely to have any more impact on health than a pinprick on the hide of an elephant is an absurd notion.

The motivations of workers engaged in such activities are, of course, not questioned. Such workers are genuinely intent on providing the individual with some control over factors that may threaten his or her health. But by creating the illusion that such factors are controllable in this way, these programmes may in fact increase the feeling of powerlessness among their client groups. The problem of illhealth is addressed by time- and energy-consuming, often costly, personal strategies. The prevalence of disease in society remains unchecked. People will still get sick, but added to their sickness will be a burden of guilt that they should have been able to prevent their illness, which, in fact, was never within their control.

Such lifestyle-oriented programmes address illness prevention in a very narrow sense. By constraining and regulating body functions and activities such programmes promise the salvation of health, and by so doing reinforce the status quo. Although the activities of such agencies are seen by many people to offer an alternative practice to clinical medicine, they are in fact synonymous with the logic of mainstream medicine. The methods may appear different, but the ideas about illness causation and location are identical. Hence such programmes reaffirm the underlying framework of medicine, and by their seeming extension beyond the central preoccupation of conventional medicine with curing, demonstrate to society a responsibility to prevent disease as well.

In its broadest sense, illness prevention is not a medical problem at all. Health is a product of the socio-economic structure of society. Town planners, road designers, food manufacturers, law makers and local governments may have a much more significant role to play in illness prevention than doctors. To make an impact on the problem of illness, attention must be directed at intervention in the socio-economic organisation of society itself (Russell and Schofield, 1986:134). Medicine, of course, should continue to play an important role, but only as part of a more genuine, thoroughgoing approach to the identification of illness causation and alleviation of the more substantial structural influences on health.

Medicine is still an extremely powerful institution in our society. Medicine has the power to define health, and to define non-health or disease. The reality defining authority of medicine is reinforced by legal sanctions expressed in medical registration boards, and by substantial social sanctions (Hicks, 1979:202).

Critical to the scientific paradigm of biomedicine is its breastplate of objectivity. Medicine is a value-free science. Diseases exist naturally and await medical discovery; such discovery leads to their explanation and subsequent control by a plethora of medical interventional strategies. Such claims to objectivity presuppose that medicine is asocial, that medicine is a body of knowledge independent of society, uninfluenced by social forces. Clearly, this is not so. Just as the body cannot be known to us except by the classificatory systems of biology, anatomy and physiology, medicine also creates health and illhealth by its classification systems. All medical categories are socially-constructed categories, categories that define and give meaning to certain classes of events. Medicine is a form of social practice, which through observation and classification provides a set of rules for viewing bodily states and conditions. As a social construction it is firmly tied to time and place, and reflects a particular way of viewing the world (Morgan, Calnan and Manning, 1985:29). Such world views are not neutral. Foucault (1973) suggests that anatomy should more properly be called 'political anatomy' since it reflects a view of the body that is congruent with the interests of dominant power groups in society. Similarly medical knowledge is never neutral. The changing nature of its categories, the non-universal characters of its beliefs and the moral underpinnings of its injunctions clearly indicate its social nature and its domination by powerful interests.

Research into health suffers from the bias of its most common starting position—the biomedical model (Freidson, 1970:260). It thus looks backward at the individual from its own normative conceptions, which arise from illhealth, not health. The self-conceptions of health, and illness, in the minds of the members of society are underrated. Assumptions that these ideas are no more than lay reflections of medical wisdom, 'folk' assessments of the situation that require medical validation, must be subjected to critical analysis. Conceptions of health are partly individual personal ideas; they are also partly socially constructed in conjunction with other people, and they are real. They must be investigated in their own terms.

The notion that the Western medical model provides the only source of rationality about health and illness must be suspended. A decision to seek medical aid is not necessarily rational action. Investigation must focus on a person's own ideas of health and illness; the rationality or irrationality of his or her action must be assessed in terms of these rather than measured in terms of the external logic of Western medicine. Medicine is but one rationality among many institutional rationalities. A person's decision to eschew outside help of any kind and engage in self-remedial action from trivial to large scale, or even to ignore illhealth altogether, may be no less rational.

Whether the conceptions people hold are accurate in any scientific sense is irrelevant. In social action analysis that which is thought to be real is taken as real. Analysis of the way ideas of health are used in social action will transform the commonsense, unproblematic notion of health into a critical concept.

Social action is action that takes into account the existence of others. It involves understanding and interpreting the meaning of another's behaviour. It is also influenced by past action and involves predictions (Schutz, 1972:144). Cultural understandings and typifications of health and illness suggest appropriate action to be taken. People's conceptions of health become visible when they are raised in social action. At what point can a person no longer take his or her health for granted? When a person's health is challenged, action may be taken. The criteria used in the assessment that either outside help or self-remedial action is needed are of crucial importance in the determination of what, in an individual's self-conception, constitutes health. An examination of these criteria can also illustrate the influence of certain cultural forms and practices in a particular individual's conception of his or her own health.

People who seek outside help are those people who see their health to be deficient. This point is important, for it presupposes an inestimable number of people who may or may not be healthy in officially understood terms, but who do not see their own health as a problem. Social action, especially in the form of appeal to social institutions or cultural practices, is triggered by a factor in the person's self-conception of health. Although this is developed in relation to others, and in a social context, it is nevertheless unique. Official statements about 'the health of the community' are ambiguous. At best they can only refer to the health of those people who seek help from one particular agency because they see some elements of their health to be a problem at one particular time (Zola, 1973:686).

Perception of illness and acknowledgement of disease involve specialist and non-specialist knowledge. Medical discussions of disease neglect the complex process of illness definition in which people engage in the everyday world before reaching a decision to seek (or not to seek) medical help. This process, though invisible to official medical agencies, is crucial to the question: what is disease? Not only does it presuppose an inestimable number of people with illness symptoms who do not see these cues as remediable by a medical agent, but it places the medical diagnostician very much in a secondary place as a definer of illhealth and disease. The individual is the definer of his or her own illhealth. The authority of medicine in our society is such that it obscures this important issue. Cultural typifications are heavily interlaced with medical wisdom. Yet an individual decides that his or her symptoms require help entirely outside the formal practice of medicine. Medicine generally sees only those people who see themselves as susceptible to its ministrations.

Most studies of the way people view illness have focussed on whether these views coincide with professional views. Quite different processes are used in lay and professional conceptions of health and illhealth, and each may be irrelevant to the other.

Fabrega's attempt to correlate scientific and native frames of reference about illness in Zinacantan supports this contention (1971). An individual may base a decision that he or she is ill on factors that a professionally trained person would find irrelevant to the specialist model. Similarly, institutional measures to improve health may fail because people do not perceive such measures to be related to their own conceptions of health. Ideas about health and disease are not the sole possession of the medical profession. While dominant, medical assumptions do not obliterate the capacity of the human mind to hold other opinions.

Early research into illness behaviour remained embedded within the medical paradigm, and thus tended to have a very individualistic bias. In contrast to such 'muddle-headed client' studies of people's responses to illness, I have attempted to highlight the complicated cognitive and interactional processes involved in the interpretation and management of signs and symptoms. My focus is on how people interpret and make sense of their own bodily disturbances—a decision to seek medical care being one option amongst a number of alternative choices that they may make. The process of becoming ill, and subsequently of becoming well are by no means as clear cut as medicine would have us believe.

Health is indeed, an elusive concept. To strive towards some idealised goal of health may be a dangerously obfuscatory activity. Health and illhealth are far too complex for simple reduction, or for simple prescriptions for attainment or alleviation. Health, and similarly, illhealth are socially constructed categories, responsive to social anxieties and concerns as well as to powerful interest groups within society.

Health is not just good luck; illness is not fate—nor are such states the outcome of moral turpitude and social degeneracy. Health and illhealth are firmly located in the socio-economic organization of society. Such knowledge brings hope, since it points clearly to the possibilities for change. Narrow definitions will handicap us in our quest for personal and social solutions to good health and the alleviation of illhealth.

4 What is disease?

Disease involves changes in the function, appearance and movement of the body, and pain. The idea of disease evokes associations of discomfort, pain and inconvenience. 'Cutting teeth', as the term implies, is an event associated with pain and discomfort, yet we do not consider this to be disease since we see it as a natural, normal process. Similarly, many women experience great discomfort, inconvenience and pain during pregnancy and childbirth. Such experiences, however, would never be seen as disease, but rather as a necessary part of the normal process of procreation. Binding the feet of upper-class Chinese women involved pain and deformity, yet this practice was not considered to be disease since it was the means of attaining the desired goal of social status in that culture. All of these events involve considerable change in function, appearance and movement of the body, and often great pain. Yet these conditions are not diseases. What is and what is not disease relates to the social ascription of what is normal, rather than to the physiological processes that may occur or to the reactions a person might have to those bodily processes. Disease has no reality in its own right: the word gains meaning only through social definition and usage. Disease is socially defined as abnormality, deviance and difference.

Witches and demons, curses and spells have long been impuned in disease causation in non-western societies. Such agencies seem bizarre to our logical western minds, yet over time many similarly exotic explanations have been given to account for disease in our own society.

The humoral theory, discussed in chapter 3, was a wonderfully integrated explanatory framework linking the body, the emotions, and at least the physical environment in an interconnected relationship. That it survived for some seventeen centuries is testimony to its explanatory and methodological success. Its broad perspective accounted for many of the contributory elements included in the modern day social perspective of illness causation. Although the humoral theory did not specifically include socio-economic or political environments as sources of disorder, the logic of balance between body, mind and environment on which this theory was based could be broadened to include such considerations without violence to its underlying principles.

This long period was followed by a stage when a variety of approaches and beliefs about disease coexisted. In general though, perspectives up to the late eighteenth century tended towards a very individualistic focus. Disease resulted from an underlying state of the body, but the individual provoked the flowering of disease by his or her state of mind.

The nineteenth century brought a major paradigmal shift in ideas about disease causation. The work of Louis Pasteur in identifying the relationship between microbes and disease, and the subsequent work of Pasteur's German colleague Robert Koch in relating specific microbes to the causation of specific diseases were the major catalysts to a radical new way of conceptualising disease.

The germ theory of disease, and its logical successor, the doctrine of specific aetiology, brought major changes to understanding about illhealth and disease. Illness could now be pinned down, located, positively identified with a particular disease organism. Environments, temperaments and humours could now be cast aside as sources of disease causation. Witches, demons and evil spirits could no longer strike terror into people's hearts. The mind as the site of wrong thinking, evil machinations and distorted perceptions could be disregarded as a source of bodily disturbance. Disease was clearly and unequivocally caused by germs. The task was to locate the specific disease causing organism, and having identified it, the disease could be treated.

The clinical task became a sequence of fitting the patient's symptoms into a specific disease category through observation, physical examination and various strategies for the measurement of internal bodily processes. The discovery of the stethoscope in 1819 allowed the doctor access to a person's heart and lungs, the sphygmomanometer tapped the privacy of the circulatory system. Such simple devices laid the technical basis of diagnostic scientific medicine, and were the precursors of today's highly sophisticated body scanners.

The specific nature of disease causation led, logically, to a view that disease was universal. Specific causative agents would be expected to produce similar symptoms and processes, and respond in a predictable fashion to an established intervention strategy. Disease was seen as a universal category—it held its constancy across class, gender and ethnic boundaries and through time.

The liaison of germs and science to form the monocausal model of disease led to a perception of the body as a machine—a loose collection of parts, each of which could be examined and worked upon separately without the rest of the body being disturbed. But the marriage of germs and science also provoked the divorce of the body from its previous partnership with the mind. The body and the mind were no longer connected. A person's feelings, emotions and understandings no longer had to be accounted for in the difficult task of disease identification; such subjectivities would no longer get in the way of solving the body's problems. The cause of illhealth resided in the individual's body. Neither the world out there, nor the mind in here warranted consideration. A disease was a disease was a disease, located squarely in the individual. Amelioration of this undesirable state focussed on interventionist strategies directed at the body, either by stimulating the body's normal resistance to specific disease-causing agents through immunisation, or by confronting the invader head on at the time of attack through antibiotic warfare.

The isolation of specific disease-causing organisms led to the creation of the aseptic milieu necessary for successful surgical intervention. Although the discovery of anaesthesia is lost in dispute and rival claims, its clinical use was established by Yorkshireman John Snow, who administered chloroform to Queen Victoria in 1853 at the birth of Prince Leopold. Increasingly sophisticated strategies of anaesthesia enabled surgery to develop to the degree of technical excellence it has achieved today. The clinical use of x-rays, though not discovered until 1895 by Wilhelm Conrad Röntgen, added a vital element of precision to diagnosis and management of those parts of the body beyond range of the naked eye.

The interventionist perspective of modern medicine has developed from these innovative antecedents in relatively recent times. Pasteur's most significant work was in 1887, a little over a century ago, but antibiotics did not come into general therapeutic usage in Australia until the 1940s. Anaesthesia, though providing a major breakthrough in the possibilities of surgery, was not considered reliable until relatively recently. X-rays have been freely used since the beginning of this century, more freely used than was later considered to be wise.

What is disease? 41

These were the major discoveries that led to the paradigmal change and subsequent establishment of the scientific basis of modern medicine. This, a recent phenomenon, suited a particular state of socio-economic development. The reductive focus on the individual, the mechanistic approach of fixing parts of the body, and the relentless search for more and more ways of penetrating the body to unlock its innermost secrets have led to this particular formation. The tenets of such practice are interventionist and functional. Highly sophisticated diagnostic technologies probe the depths of the unknown to support physical observations and clinical judgements. Complicated chemical agents suppress, reverse or replace the action of bodily biochemistry, stimulate the electrical circuits of the heart or destroy tumorous growth. Surgery may reroute blood supplies, rearrange internal pipes and tubes, realign bones or replace entire organs with synthetic or cadaver substitutes.

Many people would consider that the most significant triumph of medicine has been the control of infectious diseases. The dramatic decline in death rate at the end of the nineteenth and beginning of the twentieth centuries was due to the reduction in mortality from infectious diseases, such as smallpox, tuberculosis, cholera, diphtheria and dysentery, attibutable to medical intervention. The work of McKeown (1979) refutes this. He claims that the reduction in mortality due to these infections can not be attributed to medicine since the drugs for suppression of these conditions and the immunisation campaigns for their prevention did not come into common usage until the major impact of these infections had been controlled.

McKeown claims that nutrition was the major determinant in the control of infectious deseases. Environmental factors such as better sanitation and cleaner water were critical, as was encouragement to limit family size to ensure that the growth of the population did not outstrip the food supply. Thus Mckeown challenges this claim to medical victory. His identification of social, environmental and behavioural changes suggests that medicine played a very limited role in the decline of mortality due to infectious diseases over the last century.

Similarly, today's major scourges—heart disease and cancer— may also relate to environmental, social and behavioural determination, and in the same manner be beyond the ambit of medical modification, except in their end-state manifestation. True prevention, as discussed more fully in chapter 3, will not be achieved by individualistically focussed behaviour change and health education programmes, although they may play a part, but by a much more wholesale approach to social inequalities, hazardous work environments and illness-producing neighbourhoods in the wider society.

Medicine itself can be incriminated as a source of illhealth and disease both directly by iatrogenesis (Illich, 1975) but also by its vested interest in the perpetuation of the prevailing paradigm and the professional structures that have arisen out of this.

Immunisation programmes, as well as antenatal screening, pap smears, glaucoma testing, community blood pressure testing and similar activities designed to detect early signs of disease-producing factors are important strategies, as are the lifestyle-oriented programmes discussed before. But these strategies represent a very limited approach to prevention—they may at best close the stable door just as the horse decides to amble out. They may enable treatment to be begun earlier, but rarely do they actually prevent disease even in the individual, let alone act on the agents of disease in the wider community. Such an approach will require attention beyond the health care sector.

Certainly some modifications have occurred over time that have added considerable breadth to the former narrow conceptions of disease. A multicausal model posits that a person's health and illhealth are connected not only to the way a person experiences his or her world but also to the way the social environment influences the individual. Social and environmental factors are considered along with clinical evidence in diagnosis and management plans. The dominant approach, however, continues to be individualistic, disease oriented and antidotal in nature. The power of medicine as an explanatory system of disease causation, as an interventionary mechanism for symptom alleviation and as a substantial structural institution of dominant ideas, values and authority remains.

The manner in which groups of practitioners gain closure, peer review, autonomy and other basic requisites for professional status, and the measures by which such groups maintain their power and defend their right to such authority from the challenges of others requires a much more thoroughgoing analysis than this work allows. Sufficient to say that even if in the face of such dominating ideas people could see the existence of a broader and more powerful explanation for disease and its amelioration, such enlightenment would not blow away the substantial social structures that have arisen and prospered under the aegis of biomedicine. Enlightenment is seldom a match against vested interest.

Medicine is a wonderfully successful paradigm—a triumph of ingenuity, creative technology and great skill. It has achieved great success in a very short time. The problem for us all is that the successes and triumphs of this paradigm have obscured the real cause of disease in society, and have prevented us from seeing more appropriate sites for intervention. By locking us into a perspective of the body as a finely-tuned machine, susceptible to invasion by organisms, wear and tear on moving parts, clogging and blocking of tubes, misrouting of synaptic messages and drying up of essential secretions, we have been seduced into reliance on this technically complex but theoretically simple model of disease causation and remediation. The objectively demonstrable successes of this model have led us to think of illness in a narrow and fragmentary manner, to neglect the enormous 'web of illness causation'.

Attention to such a perspective may have a high personal cost. Such attention would compromise our faith in our own biomedical salvation and deliver us into what must appear to be a much less comfortable paradigm. Since we shall all get sick, since we all shall die, it is not hard to see that challenging such an established reality will sow the seeds of doubt in our own inevitable dependence on biomedicine at some stage in our own lives.

A broader social perspective of disease, incorporating as it does a consideration of the social, economic and environmental determinants of disease, will not obliterate the need for the interventionist strategies of biomedicine. It must, however, shatter the complacency of our conception of the body as a machine, isolated and detached not only from the world, but from its own perceptual centre and our confidence that chemical, surgical or physical intervention can have any significant impact on the wider problem of disease in society. Because our attention is focussed on the undeniable successes of medicine, we do not see the large penumbra of illness, disease and suffering for which this paradigm can offer no solution.

The objective–subjective dichotomy is a prevailing theme, and a continual source of tension, within the biomedical paradigm. Disease, as we can see, has no objective reality, yet biomedicine is based on the recognition of objective signs and symptoms of disease—universal and timeless features of established disease syndromes. Data on temperature, blood pressure and respiration provide solid, factual, quantitative evidence and the confidence that the condition is firmly grounded in objective reality. Objectivity is the cornerstone of medicine. Yet how can such objectivity be achieved? Not only is disease a socially-constructed category, but the subjects of this objective practice are people.

The doctor comes to the medical intervention with all the objective underpinnings of that profession. The doctor deliberately sets his or her vision to the tunnel mode, expressly sees only clinical signs and asks only about medical symptoms. The client comes to the interaction as him or herself, with an individual's worries and concerns, interests and values. Such things cannot be left behind in the cloakroom with the umbrellas while the medical work is being done. They are integral to the person and to the meaning of the symptoms the person is bringing to the doctor.

Subjectivity is vigorously routed out of medical domains. Medical houses are routinely scoured to make sure no random subjectivity has crept in under the doors or though a crack in the window frame. Yet, of course, doctors do attend to these personal and social variables. Their insistence on objectivity, however, means that such variables are dealt with in an informal and unsystematic way that not only denies their critical importance in disease causation, but can lead to discriminatory practices. Major decisions can be made on the basis of an unacknowledged deferrment to just these factors, which officially are given so little significance. Small, largely unaccountable sections in the patient's case notes refer to 'psycho-social factors' or 'subjective examination'—often a short compendium of unthinking stereotyping and prejudice rather than any true enlightenment about the influence of such factors in disease causation or the possibilities of rehabilitation. Treatment decisions are embedded in class, age and gender assumptions; lifestyles are searched for diagnostic leads. Ethical dilemmas abound, yet all but a few masquerade as sound, clinical judgements.

Doctors' disease-focussed medical training does not prepare them for the fact that diseases come embedded in people—surrounding that disease, enclosing it, enveloping and sometimes obscuring it is a person, a person with a biography, with feelings, interests and values, with a class, age, gender and ethnicity. Not only may the person present to the doctor symptoms that do not have medical relevance, but he or she may neglect to mention symptoms that do.

Why does Mr X keep talking about his problems at work, his

worries with his wife, the trouble his adolescent kids are getting into? If only Mr X would stop talking about these things, the doctor could get down to the examination, diagnosis and treatment sequence, and solve the problem. The doctor knows that there are medical solutions for Mr X's problem, but so many issues seem to crowd in, to obscure the problem that the doctor may never get a chance to prove this point.

As the doctor becomes more familiar with the practice of medicine, he or she will learn how to control these issues which seem to crowd the medical intervention. The doctor will become much better at managing the interaction, allowing just enough subjectivity to construct a pleasant working relationship, but not so much that is obstructs the interaction.

Controlling the personal and intimate in medical encounters is a continual source of tension. Gynaecological examinations are obvious domains for dangerous assertions of the personal. Joan Emerson's study (1973) provides interesting insights into the manner in which definitions of reality are managed in this difficult context. The management of pregnancy also holds the potential for danger, but seems to be less volatile, maybe because the foetus can be used to focus the anxieties of both the doctor and the mother onto a more objective, third person.

Long-term disability, especially the type of disability that is the focus of this study can be an extremely difficult context for the management of subjectivity. To learn about the patient's former life, interests, values and potential can lead to an overwhelming feeling of sympathy for the patient. On the other hand, to ignore such personal information is to deny the client an understanding of the extent and meaning of his or her loss.

Rapprochement between scientific thinking and popular thinking will not be achieved, however, by the mere act of a doctor asking patients how they feel about their illhealth. The problem cannot be solved by such superficial strategies; it is not just about communicational difficulties, but represents a major paradigmal difference in thinking. The doctor and the patient inhabit quite different worlds; neither may realise just how discrepant these two worlds are. In a sense doctors lose their contact with the non-medical world when they graduate. Medical training is so thoroughly embedded in the internally consistent logic of biomedicine that this paradigm comes to dominate its students' thinking.

The dénouement comes, however, when it is the doctor who becomes sick. No longer can the subjective be held off; because now it is the doctor's body that feels, the doctor's own mind that thinks, the doctor's own concerns that crowd the issue. Although many articles in medical journals document the lack of control and confusion experienced by the doctor-become-patient, the work of Oliver Sacks, particularly *A Leg to Stand on* (1986), in which he documents his dilemma as both experiencer and doctor-observer of his own disease, is a particularly insightful study.

The practice of objectifying the body leads to a disembodied conception of self—a separation of the body from the self. Disease that entails a loss of self is the most proximate and universal form of human estrangement (Turner, 1984:234). Ironically, it is the very breastplate of medicine—its insistence that it is an objective and value-free science—that is the source of its major problem. This reductive perspective eliminates from consideration all those factors that make a body human, a perspective which, if unmodified, must ultimately contribute to its own demise.

Medicine does what it does well. We are to blame when we expect it to provide solutions for which its individualistic disease-focussed framework has not prepared it. But medicine fails when it leads us to believe that it can provide a solution to illness and disease in society.

We spent a considerable time in chapter 3 exploring people's self-definitions of health and illhealth. We saw that the individual may engage in a huge range of negotiations, interpretations and choices before deciding that he or she is not well, and what action, if any, might be the most appropriate to take. We saw that going to a doctor was far from taken for granted. Medicine sees only those people who see themselves at this particular time as susceptible to its ministration. The choice to 'go to the doctor' will, however, incorporate a certain view of the disease and the person, as well as dictate a particular methodological approach.

This is not to say that the person is totally committed to the logic of medicine because he or she has chosen to go to the doctor rather than a naturopath or a chiropractor. Although the individual may engage in a wide range of cognitive, interpretive and negotiative processes before going to see a doctor, this choice must not be seen to represent a free selection between a range of equal options.

In our society the profession of medicine is part of the socio-economic structure of society. Going to the doctor can be seen as the easiest choice a person can make. There is a doctor on every corner, a clinic or hospital in many suburbs and towns. Many workplaces and residential institutions have their own doctors, or if not, a health officer who will promptly refer the person to a doctor. In general, consulting hours are liberal, and reflect the established need in the area. Casualty departments in large hospitals cater for emergency problems, or those health disturbances that occur after office hours. Universal health insurance, such as Medicare in Australia, which is levied from wages, guarantees a minimum standard of treatment to everyone free of costs at the time of intervention. Moreover, medicine documents entry and exit from many roles and positions in society. Births and deaths require the legitimation that can only be provided by medicine. Certification of illness, and the medical legitimation of bodily damage and subsequent rehabilitation after injury or accident are written into the work and legal practices of society. Thus going to the doctor can be seen as the obvious, easy and responsible choice to make when faced with disturbing symptoms. To do otherwise may well be inconvenient and costly, but more importantly, may incur social disapproval.

The sudden and serious nature of the conditions that are the focus of this study, however, severely restrict the choices available. In the rest of this chapter we shall explore in more detail the medical processes that transform the person into a patient.

The stock of knowledge of medicine serves to determine and order actual situations (Schutz and Luckman, 1973:237). But relevances determine the constitution and structure of the stock of knowledge. The stock of knowledge is composed of typifications. A type is a meaning context established in experience (Schutz and Luckman, 1973:230). Typifications are elements of knowledge related not to specific objects and persons, but rather to typical aspects and attributes of objects, persons and events (Schutz and Luckman, 1973:143). Definitions of new situations are determined with the help of a type constituted in prior experience. This system of relevances and typifications functions as a scheme of orientation for each member of the medical profession, and constitutes a universe of discourse among them (Wagner, 1970:120).

The first step in the medical intervention in the illhealth of a person is to establish a diagnosis. A diagnosis is a definition of the situation, a description of a person's signs and symptoms in the language of medicine. By making a diagnosis, a doctor ascribes a label to a person's understandings of his or her own health. The process of diagnosis employs the system of medical relevances and typifications to transfer unique, individual feelings into typical features of typical medical roles (Wagner, 1970:120). By labelling and naming, the doctor relates a person's signs and symptoms on the basis of their typicality, to other signs and symptoms of similar typical structures. Identification is based on a generalised knowledge of the type of these objects, or of the typical style in which they manifest themselves (Wagner, 1970:117ff).

If the patient's signs or symptoms are recognised by the doctor as familiar, typical elements of a particular illness syndrome, the doctor applies his or her stock of knowledge in an automatic way to produce a diagnosis. This specialist knowledge acts as a template of expectations and assumptions about the disease and its future prognosis. If the presenting signs or symptoms appear less typical, the ascription of a diagnosis is less automatic. Yet processes of explication can be evoked in which new typifications are rendered familiar (Schutz and Luckman, 1973:146).

A diagnosis legitimates the understanding of a person that he or she is not well, and elevates this understanding to the status of a disease. The person becomes a patient. Ascription of a name legitimates the patient's conditions with reference to the typifications of x disease contained in the diagnostic framework of the medical specialist.

Such legitimation has social implications in the everyday world. Once feelings become detached from individual understanding, they become socially objectivated, an accessible component of the social world. Subjective understandings become objective disease—for all to see. This process sets the scene for the manner in which others perceive and act towards the patient.

Language is a system of typifying. The language of medicine corresponds to the typically relevant ideas dominant in that domain. It also corresponds to the set of types included in the stock of knowledge of members socialised in that domain. It does not, on the other hand, correspond to the stock of knowledge of most people in everyday life. Although cultural knowledge is heavily interlaced with medical wisdom, the labels, typifications and explanations of the medical domain are not part of everyday knowledge. The highly specialised language of medicine can lead to the development of a bilingual situation where one language is used about the patient and his or her condition, the other between the patient and the doctor. For the patient, the problem is a cough that keeps her husband awake at night and makes him late for work in the morning. For the doctor, the problem is pulmonary oedema. The latter has restricted meaning. The former has wide potential for ambiguity (Murrell and Barker, 1980:ch.7).

Application of the diagnostic framework of the medical domain is thus, in this sense, relatively independent of the wider social context. It can become a point of reference for the individual and others, uniting diverse explanations and contradictory understandings into a consistent whole (Kapferer, 1979:ch.4). The medical frame is a point of reference by which the understandings and experiences of the formerly healthy individual are reconceptualised in terms of the understandings of illhealth, or a particular disease entity. The symptoms of illness are articulated with wider cultural concerns of the social context in which the patient lives (Kapferer, 1979). A diagnosis of cancer, for example, would articulate wider concerns about pollution, uranium, tobacco, food additives; heart disease would lead to considerations of diet, exercise and stress. Modern disease metaphors express concern for social order. They suggest profound disequilibrium between the individual and society, with society conceived as the individual's adversary (Sontag, 1979:72).

The medical model abstracts the person from the everyday world of the taken for granted, and places him or her in the meaning province of the patient. Here the meanings and understandings of the specific disease become dominant. The commonsense understandings of others come to have less significance in the face of the expert knowledge of the medical specialist. The patient becomes distanced from the everyday world, and moves into the specific meaning context of the disease. The distinction between transitory illhealth, and disease or injury involving permanent destruction has been made in chapter 1. Transitory illhealth does not involve these processes, and does not lead to transformational change.

Cultural assumptions about a particular disease process in the wider society may further distance the individual from the everyday world of health into the subculture of a patient in a world of disease. The dominant understanding that only a medical specialist in x disease can help the patient now, isolates the patient from helpful interaction of others (Young, 1976:10). For this limited time immediately surrounding the ascription of a diagnosis, the person's understanding of him or herself become more and more consistent with those of a patient. The patient's interactive world becomes smaller and smaller. Family and significant others react to the person as a patient with x disease. The individual's conception of self is transformed into something consistent with the specialist medical and cultural conceptions of this new status.

Transformation of a person from illhealth to disease is not achieved simply by passing a person through a series of prescribed procedures. The system of relevances and typifications of medicine acts on the understanding of the person and others. The specific meaning context of the disease moulds and shapes experience in a particular way, making available new meanings and understandings to the ill person. The person's former conception of him or herself as healthy may become suppressed in the face of the dominant and tightly intermeshed ideas of the diagnostic model. Others in the everyday world readjust their conceptions of the formerly healthy person in keeping with the cultural conceptions of what x disease means in a certain social setting, what events in the patient's life could have increased susceptibility to this illness, and what the chances are of returning to society as a healthy person.

If the medical diagnostic model can be made to fit the individual's conception of him or herself as unwell, disease exists— the feelings, subjective in nature, become socially objectivated. The individual may legitimately pass from person to patient.

But the individual's understanding that his or her health is threatened may not fit the ready-made medical diagnostic model. Some of the problems that may eventually be defined as relating to the disease emerge from the diagnostic and definitional process itself. The sick person and the doctor collaborate to construct symptoms appropriate to a diagnostic model (Kapferer, 1979). If the current experience is not sufficiently typical for determination and mastery of the situation, processes of explication are induced in which new typifications on other levels of determination are rendered familiar (Schutz and Luckman, 1973:146). Tests, examinations and questioning may elicit some factors, not previously raised, which may consolidate the individual's understanding into the security of a clearly defined medical model. Great elasticity may sometimes be needed to include a person's presenting symptoms as a rare, but not unheard of manifestation of x disease. Should even this be impossible, a medical doctor has no recourse but to conclude that there is no medically recognised disease, syndrome or condition to accommodate the individual's understanding of his or her health as a problem. The individual's feelings of pain and discomfort do not receive objectivation and legitimation.

Medicine is such a dominant ideology in our society that no cultural understanding can allow a person to be sick for any length of time without medical legitimation. The individual is denied the right of conceptual transformation of him or herself as a patient, and is not seen as such by others. Instead the person is labelled, by default, as a hypochondriac, a malingerer —someone imagining sickness.

Even if medical intervention defines and legitimates disease in a patient, professional conceptions of disease prognosis may not coincide with the patient's self-definition of his or her stage of rehabilitation to health, or continuing patient status. Charges that the patient is making a career of being a patient are levelled at people whose self-conceptions fail to coincide with the professionals' expected time sequence of a particular disease process.

This chapter has served several purposes. By examining different theories of disease throughout history, the changing nature of disease explanations has been exposed, the socially constructed nature of their content has been established. Many of the shibboleths of the biomedical model, particularly its claims to scientific objectivity and value-free practice, have been scrutinised.

Yet the research on which this study is based is firmly located within the paradigm which has just been questioned and destabilised. I am aware of the pragmatism of my approach, yet to explore the transformation of a person into a patient, and subsequent transformation from this social category into a healthy person again through the disease categories established by medicine will provide insights into some of the assumptions and limitations of this approach and point to areas for modification and change.

5 Rehabilitation—the challenge to medicine

Medicine does what it does well, of that there is no doubt. Matching an individual's signs and symptoms to an established disease category through processes of observation, examination and measurement involves experience and great skill. Decisions about the most appropriate intervention, and the sequence and timing of such strategies require highly expert knowledge. Medicine and surgery, anaesthetics and pathology deserve their respected positions as major practices within the paradigm of modern medicine. Other specialities, organised around different parts of the body or particular disease categories share the triumph of modern medicine.

Rehabilitation is one such speciality within medicine. The use of the term 'rehabilitation' is broad, referring to the general provision of services and allowances to certain disadvantaged groups (Rothwell:1984). The word 'rehabilitation' in this study refers to the accepted medical usage of the term: the restoration of the handicapped to the fullest physical, mental, social, vocational and economic usefulness of which they are capable. This definition, provided by the United States National Council on Rehabilitation, has wide acceptance in Australian rehabilitation circles (Thorne and Wilbe, 1987:7).

Before federation in Australia, responsibility towards people with disabilities and other disadvantages was considered to be a matter of charitable concern rather than a governmental obligation. Colonial administrators felt that direct government assistance to such people would undermine individual initiative and encourage dependency (Rothwell, 1984:5). By the turn of the century, however, the social aftermath of the gold rush of the 1850s and the economic crisis of the 1880s and 1890s forced governments to consider welfare and policy issues. Old-age and invalid pensions and maternity allowances were substantial indications of government involvement in social welfare.

The two world wars have had a major impact on the development and nature of rehabilitation, in fact the term 'rehabilitation' was probably first used in relation to the provision of assistance to servicemen after the First World War (Rothwell, 1984:1). Rehabilitation became synonymous with repatriation, at least for this time. It was obvious to governments that those people who had sacrificed themselves for their country deserved substantial acknowledgement of their sacrifice. Compensation such as pensions, medical services, vocational retraining and financial assistance for reintegration into civilian life were some of the measures by which the nation expressed its gratitude to those people who had defended its honour and integrity in times of war.

It was not until the 1940s, however, that the government provided actual rehabilitation services to the disabled; a series of acts and schemes were precursors of the Commonwealth Rehabilitation Service, which was established in 1958 (Rothwell, 1984: 12). More recently, rehabilitation was seen as the right of every citizen who has been disabled or disadvantaged for any reason. To quote the findings of the National Committee of Enquiry into Compensation and Rehabilitation in Australia, chaired by Justices Woodhouse and Meares:

> All handicapped persons have a right not only to survive and exist but to develop and affirm their personalities. This is not a luxury to be offered only when economic grounds justify it. The handicapped are entitled to all the assistance and protection which can reasonably be provided to ensure that they can find a worthwhile place in society, a sense of dignity and responsibility and, wherever practicable, be returned to work and able to engage in sporting, recreational and cultural activities. (Woodhouse and Meares, 1974:15–16)

The Committee of Enquiry also pointed out that the rights of the disabled go far beyond simple medical rehabilitation to the requirements of the whole person, including social, vocational and educational services (Rothwell, 1984:2). Thus human rights and the concept of equal opportunity for all people have been the most powerful catalysts for rehabilitation reform in recent years. Major philosophical changes such as deinstitutionalisation, normalisation and independent living have led to new directions in rehabilitation practice and outcome.

Re-entry into the workforce was the common goal of rehabilitation programmes after both wars. Retraining or redeployment of ex-servicemen and women was a realistic goal at these times since each post-war period was a time of economic boom, with the accompanying huge demand for workers of all kinds. This close association of rehabilitation with re-entry into the workforce has been a dominant theme in rehabilitation throughout most of the century, a theme that was not challenged until the beginning of the 1970s, when structural unemployment became a reality. Since then rehabilitation programmes have de-emphasised vocational training and attempted to stress that successful community reintegration does not necessarily require remunerative employment. This change in rehabilitative goal from work to meaningful lifestyle is often incompletely articulated, however, and the orientation of both professional worker and client may still be directed at these earlier vocational goals.

One hundred years ago, the categories of people requiring charitable assistance related closely to the public concerns and anxieties of the time. Thus there were homes for 'destitute women and children', 'friendless and fallen women', 'the aged and infirm' and 'old men' (Rothwell, 1984:16). The increasing influence of medicine in the welfare area was reflected in the more recent classifications of such agencies—spastic centres, home for incurables, head injuries units, geriatric centres, dementia units—though normalisation practices are currently substituting such medical labels, often with euphemisms.

Medicine has always played an important role in welfare services, but its role in contemporary rehabilitation is much more direct. Although a growing army of different professionals work in rehabilitation teams, the training of these professional workers is located largely within the medical paradigm, the team is likely to be coordinated by a doctor, and the rehabilitation plans are most often oriented around an individualistic and physical perspective. Professional workers may compete for recognition and status between themselves, but their goals for the client often represent a very similar perspective of rehabilitative vision.

Yet maybe it is here, within this speciality called rehabilitation, that the contradictions of the medical paradigm become most apparent. The wide range of services involved in rehabilitation, and the close, long-term association between client and worker challenge the ideal of scientific detachment and objectivity even more directly than the usual medical interaction. Diverse practitioners bring different ideas and values into the rehabilitative arena, which, while not antithetical, may nevertheless challenge the dominant reality. Humanitarian and idealistic principals may override the more utilitarian and functional goals of clinical medicine.

A spinal injuries unit is a highly specialised domain within rehabilitation, and within the broader profession of medicine. As the name indicates, the work of a spinal injuries unit is the rehabilitation of an individual after damage has occurred to the spinal cord either by injury or disease. The particular problems experienced by people who have become paraplegic or quadriplegic provide insights into many other conditions involving bodily change, either internal or external, visible or invisible, progressive or of sudden onset, with which men and women must come to terms. Of course, the nature of the condition, the degree of severity and the age of onset have important implications for the manner in which an individual experiences bodily alterations, and manages the changes that the condition brings to his or her life, but many elements are common to all disabilities, illnesses and diseases regardless of their nature and extent.

Poliomyelitis is now almost totally eliminated as an acute infection, although its consequences live on. Acute poliomyelitis, because of its infective nature, necessitated isolation in an infectious diseases hospital for many months. Gentle passive movement of affected muscles was begun almost immediately, but active rehabilitation was deferred until after the acute phase had passed. The person with residual severe muscle paralysis resembled a traumatic quadriplegic or paraplegic, and was rehabilitated as such.

Anticipation of muscle recovery after the disease has run its course is an important element in the recovery stages for the poliomyelitis sufferer. Although traumatic quadriplegics and paraplegics hope for some recovery after the spinal shock has passed, the chances of any actual recovery are very small. Another factor that differentiates between the two medical conditions is the infectious nature of the polio virus, requiring the isolation of the patient in an infectious diseases hospital for some time.

There are many medical conditions which lead to serious paralysis. Paraplegia and quadriplegia have been chosen because of the sudden nature of their onset. In both conditions the individual is precipitated into an unknown world. Institutionalisation is inevitable in the early care of all quadriplegic and paraplegic people. Before the Second World War, the treatment of severely paralysed people was restricted to the preservation of life. This battle, often hard won, was an end in itself. Little thought was

56 Bodily alterations

given to how the paralysed person would live the life that had been saved.

Anticipation of war casualties with spinal cord injuries precipitated the development of spinal injuries centres in England. The Stoke Mandeville Spinal Injuries Centre was developed in 1944. The object of this centre was not just to preserve the lives of paralysed people, but to give them a purpose in life. A comprehensive programme of treatment and rehabilitation, begun immediately after the injury, was initiated (Guttman, 1967:116).

Sport has been an essential component of rehabilitation since the inception of the Stoke Mandeville centre. The social and psychological consequences of participation in sport were considered equal to its immense physical benefits for the physically disabled. The first Stoke Mandeville Games took place in 1948. In 1952 these games became an international event and now are held yearly either at Stoke Mandeville or in the country hosting the Olympic Games (Guttman, 1967:125).

Reintegration into the workforce has also been a vital element of rehabilitation at Stoke Mandeville. The goal of re-entry into a satisfying occupation is pursued through many vocational retraining programmes and sheltered workshops.

This concept of congregating people into spinal injuries centres for an integrated programme of treatment and rehabilitation, initiated at Stoke Mandeville, has been the model for spinal injuries centres throughout the world. Sir Ludwig Guttman, the pioneer director of the Stoke Mandeville Spinal Injuries Centre, was the leading proponent of such rehabilitation and published prolifically on this subject in journals and books. At the invitation of governments he visited many countries to advise on the setting up and management of spinal units. His dominant influence was not diminished by his death in March 1980. Since 1954 spinal injuries units in Australia have been established in Perth, Melbourne, Sydney, Adelaide and Brisbane. With minor variations, these units closely resemble the Stoke Mandeville model (Guttman, 1973:ch.3).

The spinal cord is an extension of the brain that contains nerve cells and their fibres. Like the brain, the spinal cord is soft and easily damaged. It is enclosed within a bony yet flexible spinal column. Mechanical injury causing fracture of the spinal column may damage this sensitive structure. The cord may also be injured by poliomyelitis, a viral disease that attacks the anterior horn cells, which innervate the skeletal muscles of the body (Harrison, 1962).

Paralysis of varying degrees may result from spinal cord injury or disease. Depending on the level at which spinal cord damage has occurred, a person may become either a quadriplegic or a paraplegic. Quadriplegia is a partial or complete paralysis involving all four limbs and trunk, including respiratory muscles, resulting from damage to the spinal cord in the neck. Prior to the Second World War, almost no quadriplegic people survived, but advances in medical, nursing and rehabilitation procedures have greatly increased the life expectancy of such people. Paraplegia is a partial or complete paralysis of both lower limbs and all or part of the trunk as a result of damage to the thoracic or lumbar spinal cord or to the sacral nerve roots (Bromley, 1976).

Injury to the cord may cause more than a loss of motor power. Deep and superficial sensation, vasomotor control, bladder and bowel control and sexual function may also be lost. The spinal cord not only conveys impulses to and from the brain but it is also a nerve centre in itself. Through various afferent and efferent pathways, the spinal cord is a vital link in the control of involuntary muscle.

The level of the lesion will determine the severity of the disability; the higher the level of the lesion the greater the disablity since more muscles and sensors will be affected. The residual disability will also be influenced by the extent of the original lesion. If the lesion was complete and no nerve endings remain intact, all functions of the cord below the level of the lesion will be lost. If the damage was incomplete, part of the spinal cord below the level of the lesion will retain function. The completeness of the original lesion will thus have a significant effect on the residual abilities of different people who may be injured at the same vertebral level.

Immediately after the injury the individual is in a state of spinal shock. This depression of nerve-cell activity can last either a few days or up to six weeks. Gradually the cells of the now isolated cord recover independent function, though now no longer controlled by the brain. The heightened reflex activity of the isolated cord may increase the tone in the paralysed muscles causing spasm, which can be very disabling in its own right.

The medical management of spinal injuries involves a specially trained and coordinated team of professional workers. The director of the spinal unit is in complete charge of the injured person.

Problems with various aspects of the body are dealt with as they arise by consultation with other specialists.

Usually the paralysed person is immobilised in an acute spinal unit immediately after the injury to allow stabilisation of the fracture, with or without surgical intervention. In order to stabilise a fracture in the cervical spine, holes may have to be drilled into the skull and tongs inserted to immobilise the head along with the rest of the body (Trieschmann, 1980:11). A tracheostomy may be performed to ensure adequate respiratory function, and an artificial respirator may be necessary. Catheterisation of the bladder is instituted to ensure proper urinary drainage during the initial stages following the spinal cord injury. Liquid intake must be monitored to maintain correct fluid and electrolyte balance. Food intake must also be regulated in the initial period since intestinal and rectal function is likely to be impaired. Laxatives and digital evacuation of the bowel will be required since the risk of intestinal obstruction is high, especially with high-level lesions.

Pressure sores or decubitus ulcers present a major problem. Pressure sores result from constant pressure on prominent weight-bearing parts of the body. The patient will be turned every two hours day and night to change the pressure on the skin in an effort to prevent such sores (Trieschmann, 1980:11). Physiotherapy is an important aspect of acute care of the paralysed person. Positioning of the person to prevent overstretching of functional muscles and to avert contractures and pressure sores, and assisting the patient to expectorate mucus from his or her lungs are essential early activities.

When the vertebral fracture has stabilised, usually between six to twelve weeks (Illis, Sedgwick and Glanville, 1982:187), the second phase of rehabilitation begins. Since there is no treatment for restoration of spinal cord function, the damage is permanent. Rehabilitation is thus based on utilising the remaining intact functions and developing mechanical strategies for maintaining vital bodily activities.

The initial acute stage of spinal injury management involves intensive medical and nursing activities; things are done to and for the patient. The second phase represents a transition from these dramatic life-saving endeavours to an educational focus whereby the paralysed person must learn the activities necessary for his or her daily life. Second stage rehabilitation ideally consists of four interlocking components: evaluation, the rehabilitation programme itself, discharge planning and follow-up care

(Hirschberg, Lewis and Vaughan, 1976). Data, including information about medical history, diagnosis, physical loss and psychosocial assessment is collected so that the staff may evaluate the patient's condition and plan a rehabilitation goal.

The rehabilitation team usually comprises medical, nursing, physiotherapy, occupational therapy, social work, physical education and vocational guidance workers. Techniques of mobility and activities of daily living are taught. Instruction in using a wheelchair, learning to change position in bed to avoid pressure sores, tranferring from bed to chair and chair to bed, and, for those people with lower-level lesions, learning to drive a car with hand controls represent considerable freedom for the previously bed-bound person. Relearning the basic tasks of bathing, grooming, dressing and eating can present major personal challenges in those activites, which have been taken for granted since infancy. A new preoccupation with skin care and bladder and bowel management must take on the nature of major obsessions, since neglect has serious consequences. Only people with lesions at the level of the lowest cervical vertebrae can hope to achieve any real independence in these activities (Trieschmann, 1980:6); people with lesions above this point will be heavily dependent on family, friends, personal attendants and others for the rest of their lives.

Planning for discharge should be interwoven throughout the rehabilitation programme. Neither staff nor paralysed person should lose sight of the fact that these activities are preparations for re-entry into the real world of everyday life, not ends in themselves. Leaving the security of the spinal injuries unit to return home can be a devastating experience. Careful negotiations with all the people involved in resettlement, and painstaking preparations are needed to facilitate this difficult transition (Jones and Jones, 1975). Follow-up visits to the unit or home visits by rehabilitation staff ensure that the person does not regress once he or she has left the spinal injuries unit, that the goals planned by the institution have been maintained.

The spinal injuries unit is a highly specialised domain within the profession of medicine. Spinal units place great importance on the necessity to live an organised life with strict adherence to daily routines. Retraining of bowel and bladder function is taught by a specialist team. Mandatory physiotherapy, occupational therapy and remedial gymnastic sessions take up much of each day. Sport and vocational retraining, major facets of the Stoke Mandeville programme, are also important elements of the rehabilitation programmes in Australian units. In consultation with family and friends, the social worker negotiates a place in the outside world for the paralysed person. Informal outings, barbecues and parties are organised from time to time by different staff members. These activities are seen as adjuncts to the essential medical work of bodily restoration.

The spinal injuries unit is thus a paraplegic and quadriplegic world, a world within yet isolated from mainstream medicine, a world within, yet isolated from everyday life. Yet it is a world constructed specifically to help the person back into the non-paralysed world, the public world of action and movement, the dynamic world of values and statuses—the world in which the now paralysed person first came to know him or her self.

Rehabilitation work is work on the body; rehabilitation workers are body workers par excellence. Central to the rehabilitation task is the enhancement of residual parts of the body and the substitution by mechanical strategies and devices for those functions of the body that have been lost. The body, its organs, its surfaces and its extremities are the central focus of professional attention. Successful body work is the key to liberation. By learning to control his or her bladder and bowel, and developing new strategies to substitute for sensations and voluntary movement, the person learns how to master those activities of the body that have been cut adrift from their central regulation. It is only by intensive concentration of energy and unremitting work on the body over many months that the paralysed person will be able to re-enter the everyday world.

It is within the spinal injuries unit that the tenets of scientific objectivity and value-free practice of the medical paradigm may meet their most significant challenge. Such tenets hold that the body can be operated upon independently of the person, that intervention into parts of the body is an activity detached from other aspects of the person. With paraplegia and quadriplegia the body and the self become separated. The person's self no longer relates to the physical body that houses it, nor to the social world from which it arose. The relationship between the body, the self and society is rendered chaotic.

Yet the objective focus on the body in rehabilitation activities perpetuates and reinforces the very problem it seeks to solve. Because of his or her injuries the person, a unity of body, self and society, becomes a patient in a medical domain—a body, an entity detached from its essential identity and social context. In the institution the self is subjugated in favour of the body.

Rehabilitation workers direct their energies to the body in order that the patient may be able to leave the institution. But such pragmatism, no matter how well motivated, may have a high cost. By reinforcing the estrangement of body and self caused by the injury or the disease in their rehabilitative practices, workers create an even more profound form of alienation.

The individual focus of rehabilitation adds to this estrangement. In order to encourage the paralysed person to own their disability, rehabilitation workers stress that each person is responsible for his or her own body, that rehabilitative triumphs as well as bodily disturbances are issues located solely within the individual. Yet, as we discovered in chapter 2, the body is a social and cultural construction. We come to know our body, to evaluate its appearance and performances through socially-given categories and understandings. The paradoxical situation of being held responsible for your body, the apprehension of which is constructed in the social world beyond individual control, is another substantial contradiction embedded in the medically-oriented paradigm of rehabilitation that significantly contributes to the distress of the paralysed person.

Battle analogies are often heard in rehabilitation settings. Injunctions to 'fight the disease', to 'conquer the disability' and to 'battle against and overcome the injury' may be helpful, but they contribute to the idea that the problem is located solely within the individual. Such injunctions occlude the fact that the person has had previous conceptual and actual affiliations in his or her social world, and moreover, they assume that this world will cleave to accommodate the 'new' man or woman if he or she can overcome the injury. Such an individualistic focus obscures the fact that paraplegia and quadriplegia are body alterations— alterations to the meaning and experience of the body, which has been socially and personally constructed over a very long time and cannot now be ignored. Moreover, paraplegia and quadriplegia exist as social categories, as collections of social understandings and knowledges that come to be seen as consistent with these conditions. Such social categories will not vanish away because it suits an individual for this to happen.

On the basis of their training and experience rehabilitation staff develop sets of expectations and understandings about each level of vertebral injury or disease syndrome. Such typifications include estimations of the extent of the loss and prognoses of rehabilitative potential, often with quite precise details of what an x-level paraplegic should be able to do. Such professional constructions usually have a high degree of universality; with minor divergences most other rehabilitation workers would subscribe to a similar set of expectations and prognoses about x-level paraplegia and would base their rehabilitative efforts on this typification. These professional constructions of typicality become templates of normality for lesions at different vertebral levels. An x-level paraplegia evokes a consistent set of expectations in the minds of rehabilitation workers, as does a y-level quadriplegia. It is normal for an x-level paraplegia to do this, and to feel like that.

Such typifications of normality based on clinical criteria, however, have little meaning for the paralysed person. The paralysed person is still operating with a radically different idea of normality from the one presented by the rehabilitation team. The person's self-identity was constructed in a very different world from the paraplegic and quadriplegic one, and has little or no congruence with the construction of normality proffered by the rehabilitation worker. The staff see the person as an x-level paraplegic. The person sees himself as himself. As we shall see in the following chapters, the person gradually lets go of some aspects of his or her former construction of self on becoming a patient, but until this time the rehabilitation worker and the paralysed person operate in quite different contexts of meaning.

It is in this domain of spinal injuries rehabilitation that the value-free tenet of medicine must also be questioned. Body paralyses require long-term management in settings often set apart from the everyday world. The patients are overwhelmingly young and male (see Figure 5.1). Although such people are severely disabled, they are seldom sick, in the common meaning of the word, after the first few weeks following their injury. Physiotherapy, occupational therapy, nursing and gymnasium sessions are usually of long duration, and repeated every day or sometimes several times per day. Contradictory realities may develop in these situations. In contrast to the short-term, sharply focussed interventions of conventional medicine, the body work in such settings is likely to involve close, long-term associations with young people who are mentally alert. In these interactions the participants may get to know each other well. Such familarity is more a component of intimate relationships than medical work, in which context subjectivities and personal components are usually rigorously controlled.

Such settings involve a wide range of services and diverse workers from different educational background, class, gender

Figure 5.1 Patients discharged from Royal Adelaide Hospital with fractures of the spinal column with spinal cord injury (July 1983–July 1988)

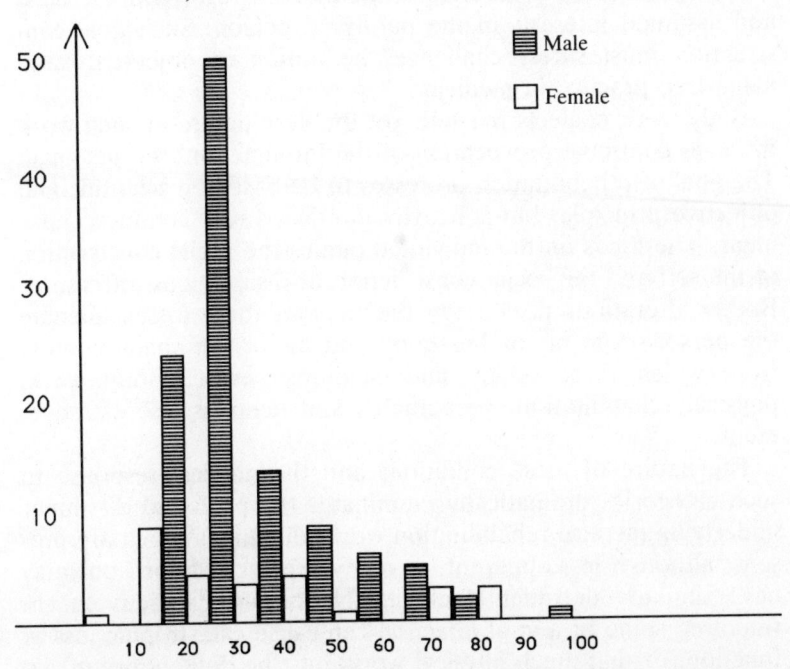

and age affiliations. Although most workers are trained within the broad ambit of medicine, in such a setting these workers may easily be tempted to abandon the rigour of this paradigm and introduce divergent ideas into the management context, an issue that will be explored in chapter 7.

The youth of the client group, and the 'it can happen to you' nature of such injuries, also engenders sympathy and empathy—an identification of the worker with the client—which may not be so usual in other medical settings. Such identification may also encourage less rigid attention to medical practice. The utilitarian and functionalist goals of clinical medicine may come into conflict with the humanitarian orientation of this specialist rehabilitation setting.

The creation of a rehabilitation goal for the paralysed person may also challenge the value-free contention of the scientific medical paradigm. Such a goal is a professional construction that evolves from commonsense theories about what will be best for this person now. This construction is based on typifications about what an x-level paraplegic should be able to do, but also on many commonsense theories related to the age, gender, class and assumed interests of the paralysed person. Such goal construction must surely challenge the notion of objectivity and value-free practice in medicine.

Body work neglects the self, yet the very nature of such work involves continual provocation of the intimate and the personal. The goal of rehabilitation professes to be based on scientific and objective principles but is heavily interlaced with common sense ideas. The focus on the individual denies the social construction of the self and the social construction of disability as difference. Bodily alterations disembody the person, these losses alienate the person from his or her body and his or her social context from which these bodily understandings arose. Body work, physical rehabilitation, perpetuates and deepens this estrangement.

The nature of these conditions and the medical response to such categories dramatically illuminates the profound dilemmas underlying medical rehabilitation work, dilemmas which are present, although less apparent, in many other conditions but may have similarly detrimental effects. No one would deny that a fractured spine or a viral infection can cause catastrophic loss of function, or that much physical work must be done in order that the individual may live and re-enter everyday life. But the energy and enthusiasm for physical rehabilitation may obscure the fact that the loss is not just a physical one, it may prevent us from seeing other dimensions, maybe more important dimensions in the rehabilitation of people with bodily losses. Such empirical rigour hides the fact that a person is a subject, not an object—and that genuine rehabilitation may be impossible within an institutional setting and may be beyond the ambit of medicine.

The logic of treatment and management of the paralysed patient in a spinal injuries unit is highly organized and consistent. The integrated team members of the specialized unit share a well-developed set of understandings about the nature of quadriplegia and paraplegia and what is to be done. Information about the patient is collated from many sources. Staff conferences, case notes and ward rounds keep each member of the team informed about the progress of the treatment. The unit is able to predict the likely outcome for each person on the basis of past experience with similar people. To the newly paralysed person, the spinal unit projects a sense of competence, experience, coordinated effort and highly expert knowledge.

Quadriplegia and paraplegia are permanent. The period spent in a spinal injuries unit is only a short time in a person's subsequent life but this time is very influential. It is within the context of the institution that the person first experiences the rupture between his or her self identity and his or her body; that the person comes to understand himself or herself as a paralysed patient.

The outlook for people suffering trauma or infection of the spinal cord has improved dramatically in the last forty years. In contrast to the former defeatist attitudes towards the treatment of paralysed people, the idea that rehabilitation is possible despite permanent physical loss is a revolutionary concept. Yet amidst the energy and enthusiasm of the rehabilitation program it is seldom considered that the real concern for the paralysed person today is not that he or she will die but that he or she may have to live.

6 Person to paralysed patient

The theoretical and analytical basis of this chapter was laid down in chapter 4. What follows is an attempt to relate this theoretical basis specifically to body paralyses. By observing the institutional imperatives and organisational factors that act to transform the person to a paralysed patient in these particular conditions, we can begin to understand the effect of such factors in many other less dramatic conditions with which men and women must cope throughout their lives, in both medical and other diverse settings.

The event

The initial onset of these conditions is usually clear and unambiguous. In the case of a traumatic injury, one minute an individual is pursuing everyday life; the next he or she cannot move, there is no feeling in the limbs. The onset of poliomyelitis is only slightly less dramatic. Often for a few days preceding the onset of paralysis, the person feels unwell, but no more than a mild headache, a few pains, a bit of giddyness—symptoms that may have been experienced before. Jim, aged 24 at the time, justified his feelings of illhealth as a Sunday morning hangover after celebrating a win at football the previous day. He realised that he had not voided his bladder for some time, so he planned a hot bath 'to get things going'. He got into the bath, but couldn't get out. Paralysis had occurred in less than five minutes.

Maggie had literally just stepped off a ship from Britain when she became paralysed. She had been feeling tired and giddy for a few days before landing, but attributed this to the upheaval of moving a family to the other side of the world. Maggie and her husband had just settled themselves and their two young children into a migrant hostel in the city when her swallowing became affected. This symptom concerned her. There had been a poliomyelitis epidemic in a nearby English village the year before in which 30 people had died. Because of her previous knowledge of the symptoms of poliomyelitis, the diminution of her ability to swallow was for Maggie a cue that she must seek help. So within three days of arrival in Australia, Maggie found herself in a large general hospital in the city. The paralysis inexorably developed over two days, accompanied by a loss of respiratory function and a continuing difficulty in swallowing.

Bob was twenty years old and, like Jim, extremely physically fit when he contracted the polio virus. Although he had not been feeling well for several days, he was used to ignoring these symptoms of illhealth. A high temperature provoked him into going to bed early. He woke up next morning totally paralysed.

Diagnosis

The dramatic and highly visible nature of the symptoms in paralytic poliomyelitis and spinal injury usually lead to a clear and early diagnosis. The diagnostic model acts as a template of expectations and assumptions both for the staff and for the individual. The medical label quadriplegia or paraplegia immediately propels the individual into a specialised institutional treatment trajectory (Strauss, 1975). A closely articulated set of ideas about what is to be done is initiated, based on the staff's past experiences of typical cases (Schutz and Luckman, 1973:243).

A clinically ascribed diagnosis legitimates the understanding of a person that he or she is not well, and elevates this understanding to the status of a disease or a syndrome. The process of diagnosis employs the system of relevances and typifications of medicine to transfer unique, individual 'feelings' into typical functions of typical medical roles (Wagner, 1970:120). Within this frame a person's conceptions of his or her health can be rearranged in order to be reconceptualised as a self-conception of a quadriplegic or a paraplegic. The person becomes a patient. But this transformation of an individual's self-conception as a patient should not be taken for granted. The changed conception of self is a personal and unique process. It cannot be tied to medical time or predicted by official assessments of typicality.

The medical model of quadriplegia or paraplegia erects a framework of assumptions around the patient. Within this frame professional, expert knowledge becomes paramount. The person becomes isolated in the world of the patient both practically because he or she is no longer a participating member of the everyday world, and conceptually by the way others see him or

68 Bodily alterations

her. The typifications and assumptions of the medical diagnostic model are of paramount importance for the staff, and thus have great influence on the patient and others. The organisational and conceptual logic of the treatment of spinal injuries and diseases is constructed on the basis of this framework of shared understandings about the nature of quadriplegia and paraplegia, and what is to be done.

The work of rehabilitation of a paralysed person is energetically pursued by professionally trained staff. But while working on paralysed limbs and organs, the staff must also interact with the incumbent of those body parts. Goffman discussed this precarious nature of 'people work' in his famous work *Asylums* (1968). The balancing of alternative realities—that of involvement and professional distance—of emotion and experience, of a personal theme with a work theme, is sometimes precarious for all concerned. Unstated cultural assumptions based on age, interests and intelligence of the patient may influence the way in which the staff can visualise the rehabilitative goal of treatment.

But the structural reality that the interaction is taking place within medically allocated space prescribes the type of interaction that can occur. The doctor and the staff are the people to make the 'best' decision now. The acceptance of the rehabilitative programme as 'the way things should be done' by the staff, but also by the patients and their families, illustrates the power of the taken for granted nature of social reality (Young, 1976:19). The implicit understandings and assumptions of the medical model demonstrate the power of the staff to control the conditions of the rehabilitation process taking place, and effectively disenfranchise the person. The person is recast as a patient—a medical entity—an object of medical work. Social structural factors may be beyond the immediate perception of the individuals engaged in interaction in a social setting. This does not mean, however, that these factors may not directly contribute to the construction of that interaction, or in fact to the constitution of the very sense that does not perceive them.

The use of a frame as an analytical device serves to define the individual to the staff and others as a patient. That the definition may not be clear to the individual at this initial stage does not alter its influence upon him or her. The diagnostic frame also determines an organisational treatment trajectory through which the individual's experiences come to be invested with meaning.

But although the conceptual use of frame serves to define the person initially, the subsequent development of 'the case', both in professional terms and in terms of its meaning for the individual, is emergent from the rehabilitation process itself. Don Handelman's analysis of the work of child-care workers in Newfoundland in important here. Handelman considers that the case is constructed in an ongoing dialectic between the phenomenal content and the ideas of the officials whose interpretations give structural form to the case (1975). A case develops through a number of phases. It is not determined once and for all. But the diagnostic framework provides the initial body of typifications, which give structural substance to the case. The fitting together of the typifications of the staff to elements of a particular instance or event, gives the impression of an inevitable path. Negotiations and interpretations are involved in this process. Legitimacy is given to the initial diagnostic frame and to the organisational and conceptual logic of the treatment of such injuries. A set of ideological typifications are invoked to define quadriplegics and paraplegics, who are then expected to exhibit evidence in support of these typifications. When such support is forthcoming, it is not treated as one approximation of the reality of the situation, but as *the* reality.

Handelman uses a phenomenological perspective to reveal the bureaucratic life world to be an arbitrary, but integrated and meaningful social construct. Elements considered relevant to the staff are put together to form patterns of meaning that give the case the appearance of 'the way it is'. Handelman exposes the interpretive dynamics that enable the case to appear in this taken for granted manner, and illustrates the construction of a case to be a function of the relevancies of the organisation. Handelman's analysis of the construction of a case by child-care workers in Newfoundland provides valuable insights into the emergent case of quadriplegia and paraplegia once the initial diagnosis has been made.

Although from the point of view of the staff, the individual became a patient at the moment the objectivated facts of the initial examination confirmed a diagnosis, becoming a patient for the individual takes much longer. In the face of such definitive medical certainty, the person's uncertainty, unawareness and unwillingness to see himself or herself as others do provokes great conflict.

Jim said he was told on about the fourth day that he was 'in a fair bit of trouble and that there was only a very slightly chance that I would ever regain the use of my legs. But it didn't mean a thing because I reckoned they were wrong anyway. I said, "you've got your opinion, I've got mine. Don't bother me with these things"'.

Although Maggie's previous knowledge about poliomyelitis left her in no doubt about the nature of her illness, it was about five weeks before she knew that she would 'not be a full person again'. No one ever told her directly, but despite the fact that a tracheostomy (an opening cut into the trachea to facilitate breathing) made communication very difficult, she set about gathering information from other people.

Bob was told almost immediately, but the revelation had little impact for him because he was still being carried along on the euphoria of the adventure. He did, however, strongly resist the patient status that the polio virus afforded him right from the start. On the first day he announced loud and clear, 'I am not going to be called a patient. I have a name, and I am somebody. You will refer to me as such'. Bob also objected to the fact that although he had to call the staff by their occupational titles, the staff called him by his first name. 'I am pleased that you call me Bob, but that means that means I will call you Ann, Jill or Bill. If I have to call you Nurse..., Dr..., or Miss..., you will refer to me as Mr Green. I realised very early that it was necessary to establish my own position. It was very important to keep my mind together. As time went by I played games like this with even more purpose and earnestness. I felt I had to fight to have an independent thought.' Fully realising that he had only his mind to fight with, Bob was nevertheless able to circumvent the nurses intention to shave off his beard. I said, 'No way; that's part of me and that stays there!' Bob's stand may be equated with Goffman's 'secondary adjustment', which 'provides the inmate with important evidence that he is still his own man, with some control of his environment; sometimes a secondary adjustment becomes almost a kind of lodgement for the self, a churinga in which the soul is felt to reside' (1968:56).

Jim, like Bob, acted immediately to hold off the patient status he felt the staff were determined to give him. He remembers that people were 'behaving stupidly around me. People were treating me like an object; they were not thinking of me as a person. If keeping my cool means yelling at you, then that is what I am going to do'.

Pam was a highly competitive sportsperson, as was Jim, before her car accident. Although she had not even heard the word before it became personally appropriate, paraplegia was a word she instinctively did not like. 'I was not going to be a paraplegic. I was going to beat it. I would not call myself a paraplegic!'

But the enormity of the disability in these conditions makes total rejection difficult. The individual is able to hold off some aspects of the status, but the severity of the symptoms and the assumptions of the staff and others makes this task difficult, often impossible.

A narrowed world

The medical model abstracts the person from the everyday world and places him or her in the world of the patient. Here the meanings and understandings of the specific disease or medical condition become dominant. The commonsense understandings of others come to have less significance in the face of the expert knowledge of the medical specialists. Others in the everyday world readjust their conceptions of the formerly healthy person in keeping with cultural conceptions of what poliomyelitis, paraplegia and quadriplegia mean in a certain social context; what event in the patient's life could have increased his or her susceptibility to this condition; and his or her chances of returning to society as a healthy person.

Mead argues from the position that society is prior to the individual; that the construction of a self is emergent from the interactive insertion of the individual into his or her social world. But the self is not a fixed entity, it is constantly evolving and changing. A change in a person's self conception can result from a change in a person's position in society. As a person moves from one status to another, his or her self-conception will change, as will the conception of the person by other 'significant' people, whose opinions and support are important for the maintenance of the person's self-conception (Mead, 1934:309–10). As his or her situational environment and resources change, the individual must sustain the self-conception in relation to his or her new situation or develop another self. A new self is developed by the process of interaction with significant others.

Although the infectious nature of poliomyelitis has serious consequences for the patient's relationships with others in the outside world, non-infectious, spinally-injured patients may also suffer severe dislocation of normal interaction. The person's understanding of himself or herself becomes more and more consistent with that of a patient. The arena of interaction becomes smaller and smaller. Family and significant others react to the person as a patient, although for them too the full significance of this status will take much longer to establish. Former components of the self—father, husband, cricketer, plumber—become deconstituted, collapsed into a new self, that of a quadriplegic or a paraplegic.

A transformation of meaning occurs in many former relationships. A man's self-conception as a husband, for example, is built up in the everyday world in relation to his wife and the expectations that this role brings. His self-conception will change now that he is in an institution rather than a nuclear family, now that his wife is a visitor rather than a conjugal partner. The wife may be seen by the patient to be siding with the hospital authorities rather than with her husband. Gradually the bonds between husband and wife become weaker, while the bonds between wife and hospital authorities become stronger, united in their common goal, the management of the patient.

Previous close personal and kin relationships change as these people become visitors, whose behaviour is determined by a set of prescribed rules, often unwritten, about what visitors can do, what they may say, and even where they may sit. Maggie was not allowed to see her infant daughter at all for many months, and her twelve-year-old son could only come as far as the door of the ward to see his mother. Bob was allowed to see only his parents for six months.

The necessary impedimenta of the early stages of treatment of paralysed people—respirators, catheters and urinary drainage, tracheostomies, Ryles tubes (a feeding tube passing through the nose to the stomach)—visually extract the person right out of the everyday world and into an unambiguous patient status in the eyes of others.

Jim lucidly describes the alienation of normal interrelationships caused by hospital visiting. Not only does the unusual garb of a gown and mask (compulsory attire for visitors to infectious patients) make the visitor feel different, but this apparel aligns the visitor with the staff world in the eyes of the patient. A wife or a husband becomes someone else. All facial expression is hidden. Only the eyes can make contact. The change in external appearance of the patient and his or her close relations or friends, the strangeness of the ward context and the disruption of everything taken for granted in formerly close personal relationships make visiting an extremely critical time for the patient.

Uncertainty

No matter how 'typical' the patient's condition appears to the staff, for the individual the meaning of it emerges only slowly, in a manner that cannot be predicted by others. Sometimes the quadriplegic or paraplegic is the last to realise the full implications. Davis's important study of poliomyelitis notes how long it took patients to become aware of both the physical and social implications of their condition (1964:141).

A steering failure in a truck led to Frank's extensive quadriplegia. Frank claims that no one ever told him that he had broken his neck, or that his paralysis would be permanent. Although Frank realised that he was not well, he thought that he would probably have to spend a little time in hospital before he was well enough to go home to his farm. 'I was expecting to get back to some sort of reasonable condition. I didn't ask questions because I didn't realise there was a problem. I just took it for granted that I would go back to work on the farm again.' His transfer from the acute care hospital to the rehabilitation unit confirmed this belief. Unaware of the subtleties the word 'rehabilitation' has in medical parlance, Frank assumed its more literal meaning—to restore to a previous condition. Frank's lack of knowledge about his new condition had serious consequences for the way he was able to see himself. Because neither Frank nor his wife understood the permanent nature of the disabilities, Frank did not allow himself patient status. His healthy self was never fully negated either by himself or by his most significant other, his wife of twelve months. Clearly, his quadriplegic status was firmly constructed by the medical staff. But unless the individual is able to transform his conception of himself as a healthy person into a conception of himself as a paralysed patient, the reconstitution of a rehabilitated healthy self can not occur.

The uncertainty and lack of awareness of the recently paralysed person provokes conflicts with the medical staff and others with expert knowledge. But to accuse the patient of denial, of unreality, of not accepting the condition, is to miss the point. Our perceptions are influenced by our knowledge. Denial implies that the individual is in possession of a body of knowledge, experience and meaning that he or she is in the position to assess and may choose to reject. Both acceptance and denial are positive acts. Each incorporates the idea that the individual is aware of the issues involved, and can act accordingly.

But the recently paralysed person is not familiar with this new body state. As Schutz argues, meaning is built up in experience, and hence over time. Quadriplegia has no meaning for the recently paralysed person. The unusual context of the hospital renders many of the issues of everyday life irrelevant. Because the patient has not yet experienced the new physical condition in relation to former interests and concerns, he or she cannot seriously contemplate what life will be like in the future (Wagner, 1970:112). Meaning must be deconstituted for the patient, but this can only occur through experience. Meanings of the person's formerly healthy self must be confronted and proved to be inappropriate before negation can occur. And negation must occur before previously taken for granted assumptions about the everyday world can be challenged, and a new social and personal reality constructed by the individual in relation to others.

But this can only happen when it does happen for the individual. To assume that because a doctor tells a paralysed person of his or her fate in the first few days after the injury, that the person will mechanically absorb, store and use this knowledge is empirically false. Strauss in his study of dying also notes that complexity and ambiguity are not eliminated in an open awareness context where both staff and patient know that the patient is dying. The patient may 'know'—but the experience of dying as yet has no meaning for the person (Glaser and Strauss, 1965:79). Experience and meaning must be re-established anew in the individual's world. This process cannot be tied to a medical timetable or a predictable progression of awareness. New factors continually emerge to influence the construction of meaning. Elements unrelated to the original diagnostic model become part of the ongoing process, which continally emerges and changes, but endows the individual's experiences with meaning.

Very few people to whom I spoke had anything more than a very hazy previous knowledge of what quadriplegia or paraplegia actually was. Most had never known a paralysed person before, either directly or indirectly. Even those people who had seen people in wheelchairs before had no awareness that bladder, bowel, sexual function and sensation could also be involved. People enter the state of the injured with the knowledge and attitudes of the non-injured (Litman, 1962:569).

Some people are told that they have a broken neck or a fractured back. In general cultural understanding, a broken or fractured bone is immobilised for a time, but always heals. Why shouldn't the bones of the neck and back heal just like any other bone? Of course the bony damage does mend; the adjacent spinal cord, however, does not.

Other people insisted that if they had broken their neck they would not be alive. Perhaps this idea arises from childhood warnings about climbing: 'You will fall, break your neck and die!' Since the patient is not dead, as predicted, other serious damage seems inconceivable. Media stories of the 'woman in the wheelchair for twenty years, walks again', variety—usually referring to a totally different medical syndrome—further increase the difficulty for the individual to conceive any permanence in the condition.

The 'facts', no matter how loudly and clearly given to the paralysed person, have no meaning per se. To have meaning they must be related back to the person's previous self-understanding, cultural knowledge and social understanding of what quadriplegia and paraplegia mean in a particular social setting. The facts also have to be invested with meaning both negatively in terms of what the patient can no longer do, of ways the patient can no longer conceive of him or herself; and subsequently more positively in terms of what he or she can still do, of a new self.

Some paralysed people claim that they accepted their state straight away, and were seen by the staff to have done so. Others say that even after ten years they are still learning: the way they see themselves is still changing and evolving. Staff may hold 'typical' ideas about how a patient exhibits acceptance or denial. The staff, I suggest, often assume that a patient has made a good adjustment because he or she does not challenge the diagnosis and complies with the treatment programme. Typical, visible signs are taken by the staff as proof of a patient's acceptance of the diagnosis and its implications. But a transformation of experience and meanings must occur in the person's mind. This may happen quickly, but more likely the reconstitution of meaning is a long and slow process. 'Acceptance' and 'compliance', as visible symbols, prove nothing about the way an individual is able to see the situation, him or herself and in relation to others. The meaning of the diagnosis to the individual changes as the time perspective is lengthened both practically in relation to the expectations of the treatment schedule, and conceptually as the idea of 'recovery' is lengthened until it can be incorporated no more. (Davis, 1955–6; Roth, 1963). The taken for granted assumptions of 'rehabilitation' and 'cure' undergo new meanings as the treatment programme proceeds.

Knowledge that is sought, it seems, is more easily integrated into understanding than knowledge that is presented as hard facts. But to 'know' that you need to know presupposes an awareness that there is large body of knowledge, experience and meaning to be discovered. Patients often seek knowledge from the paramedical staff, domestic staff and fellow patients. Patients may sneak up on the enormity of their situation by asking relatively trivial questions of the less senior staff. Sometimes the same question is put to several different people: sometimes the question is phrased in a different way to the same person. Often medical facts cited by the doctor are broken down and personalised by the patient when talking with paramedical and domestic staff or other patients, with whom there is a more informal relationship.

From the point of view of the staff, the failure of the patient to accept the condition presents problems in terms of practical rehabilitation. The patient is expected to spend only a certain time in a rehabilitation unit. If the person can accept that there is a problem, and can direct efforts to the rehabilitation programme, time and energy will be more economically utilised. This would make the process easier for all concerned. Yet sometimes the patients is the last to know the full implications of his or her condition.

Following exploratory surgery after a car accident, the surgeon told Pam that although she had broken her back, there was every chance that she would get some recovery. He did not mention how long she could continue to hope for this though. 'I can remember I kept saying that they said I might get some recovery. There was always the thought in my mind that I might be making all this effort [rehabilitation] for no reason.' Eventually Pam (an extremely eloquent and intelligent woman) sent her husband to ask the doctor, 'Because I was sick to death of being virtually in limbo, of not knowing'. The doctor said, 'Oh, no, no way!' She did not find this revelation devastating at all; in some ways it was a relief. 'Now it meant I could say, right! this is it! I have to get on with it.'

Jim was not able to see his situation as anything more than a temporary nuisance. One day a nurse said to him, 'You are not making as much progress as we had hoped you would. We do hope some of these muscles start to work soon'. This seemingly simple statement was very important to Jim. 'I thought, "Hang on, there is something wrong." For the first time they were taking me into their confidence.' Evidence that the staff were treating him as a person with a mind was clearly very important to Jim. Jim was a top-class sportsman. Every day stories appeared in the newspapers proclaiming his diagnosis and prognosis, sometimes in highly emotional form. 'It seemed like I was reading about someone else. Why would they be bothered writing all that when it wasn't happening anyway? What a waste of time writing about all that when I definitely will be alright.'

Most people with spinal cord damage no longer feel the sensations that indicate that the bladder needs emptying. The patient must learn to interpret other 'feelings' that the bladder is full, and how to manually stimulate the bladder to empty. Bowel control is also lost. Bowel training aims to condition the patient to produce regular evacuation, at the same time every day or second day, when the patient is prepared for it. Bladder and bowel retraining is an important issue for the paralysed person, and the relearning is enthusiastically pursued by a specialist staff team. But many people find the permanent loss of these two functions almost harder to incorporate into their understanding than the fact that they will never walk again.

Pam felt fairly confident that she would be able to cope with these two functions as soon as she got home and back into her own routine. Jim placed great hope in the fact that as soon as he could stand up again everything would be alright. 'If I could just get out and sit on the lavatory, everything will be alright. Just leave me alone. I'll fix it.' Both Pam and Jim were approaching their new problems with past knowledge that was no longer appropriate to their new state. Jim eventually stood for the first time many months later, and with a huge amount of orthopedic gear. For the first time he was able to realize that the situation he had continued to project from his former state as a solution to his present state had no validity. 'For the first time I realised that what I thought would be a solution, wasn't. I thought, "This isn't me." I was scared.' From this time, Jim allowed himself to be a patient. 'I did not want to go back to being a husband or a father. I couldn't see any future outside the hospital. I was secure where I was. Everything outside became unreal. I didn't want to go back to that.'

Frank's inability to see his quadriplegia as permanent had more serious implications for his initial rehabilitation. The unfamiliarity of a city hospital for a country farmer, and the infrequency of contact with his wife and child because of the distances involved, invested his rehabilitation stage with unreality, a time out from normal everyday life. Frank never questioned that he would go back to the farm; nor was he able to conceive that anything would be different when he did. Frank's first trip home to the country was nearly eighteen months after the injury. The confrontation between his physical condition and his everyday world dramatically provided meaning for his experiences. His sexual loss was brought vividly into his consciousness on his first night at home with his wife. The need to reorder the way he saw himself became apparent for the first time. His wife also had little understanding of the problem. Accusations that Frank should have been better than he was, that he should be able to do more for himself, were beginning signs of a marriage breakdown and divorce some five years later.

About a year after this first trip home, Frank had to go to another hospital because of a medical complication. Because he had been able to build up a picture of himself in a world that had a past meaning for him, he was now in a position to see rehabilitative measures as having some relevance for his new self. Here he was taught to use an electric typewriter, and to use a pen with an arm splint attachment. 'The occupational therapist here was able to talk to me and find out my needs. She was very enthusiastic and willing. She tried to work out what I thought was important.' Although Frank had been in a wheelchair for two years, the chair had had to be pushed by someone else. The occupational therapist put some spikes on the wheels which meant that Frank could push the chair himself. 'I was no longer totally reliant on others. This meant real freedom, real liberation for the first time for two years. It opened up a whole range of possibilities for me.'

Frank is not overstating the case when he claims that the capacity to express himself in writing, and to move without help after two years represented real liberation. He claims that this kind of information was not available in the beginning. He considers that if he had had this kind of help from the start, he would be far better off today. This I challenge.

Electric typewriters, attachment arm splints, and capstan spiked wheels on chairs are fairly standard equipment for quadriplegic patients. Almost certainly these devices would have been available to Frank at the time of his initial rehabilitation some nine to ten years before. The difference then and two years later was that Frank, through his interrelations with others in his everyday world, had come to see himself as susceptible to these measures. He was now able to accept these aids as relevant to his new conception of himself, and through using them he was able to move toward a new self with a degree of freedom and independence.

New factors become woven into the situation over time. New elements emerge and change the situation as it is defined by the paralysed individual and others. The passage of time, a new social situation, the definitions of others—all play a part in the way a person sees him or herself, and the manner in which he or she understands new information and can incorporate it into a new, but ongoing conception of self.

Isolation yet loss of privacy

Cut off from the usual complex interrelationships of social life, the patient may experience great loneliness and isolation. In the midst of a busy rehabilitation schedule, surrounded by other patients and staff, a young quadriplegic man painstakingly learning to write with a pen attached to a hand splint slowly wrote—'This ward is a very boring and lonely place to be'.

Not only do the medical facts of his condition have no meaning for him, but the understandings of others toward him are full of ambiguity and uncertainty. Relationships with the staff and visitors are based on assumptions that as yet have no meaning for the patient himself. Yet, paradoxically, this enforced conceptual isolation is accompanied by a very real loss of privacy.

Privacy about the intimate and personal features of one's self is taken for granted by healthy people in the everyday world. Joan Emerson's analysis of the social interaction in a gynaecological examination has relevance for the inevitable preoccupation with the genital organs in the management of quadriplegia and paraplegia. Balancing alternative realities, a recurring issue for paralysed people and for other people with whom they interact throughout their lives, is especially critical here. To define the treatment, which has to be done as medical work, while at the same time maintaining the integrity of the patient as a person, can be difficult for all concerned. Secondary socialisation allows the intrusion of nursing staff into this area of the body to be considered 'necessary medical work'. But this understanding is constantly challenged by taken for granted primary socialisation, which interprets exposure of the genitalia as being a private sexual concern (Emerson, 1973:360). The staff must work hard to maintain the definition of the patient as a technical object in a routine medical situation. Yet defining the person as an object is an indignity in itself. This indignity can only be redressed by

80 Bodily alterations

acknowledging the patient as a person. This inherent contradiction adds to the difficulties of both staff and patient.

The stark reality of the paralysis makes the intrusion of others inevitable. The conceptual realisation that life will never again be private takes longer to accommodate. The capacity to protect oneself from the intervention of others is very limited for a quadriplegic. A low-level paraplegic can become very independent, but not totally.

Although some patients were able to take a resigned and detached attitude towards the practical help that had to be done by the nursing staff, others strongly resented the invasion of their bodies by human and mechanical agents. Jim particularly resented the bladder catheterisation, which was an inevitable part of his early treatment. He hated the tubes and bottles, the suppositories and enemas, which are inescapable tools in bladder and bowel re-education. 'Not only can you not see or feel what is being done to you (all patients are nursed flat for at least six weeks), but you are totally unable to move to protect your privacy. Your body is invaded, and there is nothing you can do about it.'

Jim's bladder at this stage was operating through a catheter draining continuously into a Winchester quart bottle by the side of the bed. A fluid balance chart rigorously accounted for all fluids taken by mouth. Friends smuggled in some cans of beer, which were consumed in haste during their visit. Jim drank so much that the cork blew off the drainage bottle. 'To see the nurse trying to reconcile the cordial, cup of coffee and bowl of soup I had had with my urinary output was incredible. This was the first time I had laughed since I arrived.' Jim's pyrrhic victory over his mechanised bladder illustrates the depth of his frustration at the medical takeover of his body.

Certainly the abrogation of privacy in such basic acts as micturition and defaecation is a devastating loss. But privacy is also denied the patient in many other areas of institutional life. For many reasons 'batch handling' can be seen as inevitable in an institution. Yet the deprivation of privacy and depersonalisation this causes some individuals should compel its organisational benefits to be closely examined. No matter how such procedures are rationalised by appeals to institutional efficiency or patient resocialisation, these processes inevitably deconstitute the self, 'even where the inmate is willing and the management has ideal concerns for his wellbeing' (Goffman, 1968:50). Communal bathing, eating and sleeping may be helpful to many people.

Certainly some patients gain valuable information about themselves by watching others tackling similar problems. But for the many people the lack of privacy is strongly felt. A healthy person is able to minimise the effects of unpleasant aspects of his or her environment by changing or avoiding them. He or she can move furniture, can avoid loud noises, unpleasant odours or harsh lights. Although paraplegics are able to push their wheelchairs away if they wish to avoid such things, this freedom is denied most quadriplegics.

Right from the early days of his hospital stay, Bob, a quadriplegic, demanded that screens be placed around the respirator. 'This was considered out of the question by the matron, and treated as quite a joke by the nursing staff. But I insisted on privacy. I felt I had to fight to have an independent thought.' Frank was also able to express his resentment about communal treatment and the lack of privacy. 'They don't really like you to have a mind of your own in a place like this. It upsets some of them to think that you don't think the same way as everyone else.'

Commonplace, private acts in everyday life—signing a bank cheque, choosing clothes, cleaning teeth, writing a personal letter, making a phone call—all must be done with the help of an intermediary. Not only are such personal acts no longer private, but the patient must accept the act as it is done by the third person. The immediacy of direct person to person interaction is lost by the imposition of an agency in such transactions.

Information

Each event in an institution is known to everyone. Even those people who do not witness an event at first hand will soon hear of it through the formal or informal information channels. Practical progress, rebellious behaviour, personal idiosyncracies, the colour of your wife's hat—everything becomes public property, open for discussion and evaluation.

Staff talk to other staff both formally at staff conferences and informally around the tea table. Staff talk with patients both formally at ward rounds, and informally in the course of treatment. Patients talk with other patients; patients talk with visitors; visitors talk with staff formally at family conferences and informally during visiting hours. Visitors discuss the patient with others in the everyday world to which he or she will return. A complex network of information develops around and about a patient, and often over his or her head.

The power of the staff to intrude into every area of the life of the insitutionalised patient reproduces and increases staff authority and power. The professional staff assume that their specialised knowledge gives them the right to make decisions on behalf of the patient, and 'for the patient's own good'. The social worker, vocational guidance officer, and other professional staff have a mandate to discuss the patient with anyone they consider relevant. These workers are free to explore and reveal any dimension in the patient's life that they feel may hold rehabilitative potential. Not only is the patient the object of the medical work, but his or her personal relationships also become objectified as the subject of rehabilitative work. The patient's ability to withhold knowledge or control information about him or herself is severely curtailed.

In order for a future that will be 'best for the patient' to be planned by professionals, a factual remake of all that is past in the patient's life is constructed through the eyes of others. Not only is his or her body no longer private, but neither are past relationships, work and school records or personal idiosyncracies. In seeking facts to construct a rehabilitation project for the patient, the social worker does not take into account the subtleties or historical dimensions of a relationship, the meanings or understandings that exist in even the simplest relationship. The medical worker is forced to take relationships at face value, often with serious consequences for the people concerned when they must interact in the medically-interpreted construction of such relationships.

Interpretation necessarily creates discrepancies between the patient's world as it is seen by him or her, and this world as it is seen by a case worker. Not only is information subject to interpretation by the donor, but also by the professional collector and later by the organisational user of the information. Handelman (1975:66) also notes this chain of information. By this time, 'impressions' and 'conjectures' have been passed into a formal conference context, and given status as facts by being written into a medical record.

A formidably detailed information network, arising from diverse sources and containing assumptions, prejudices and 'hard facts', whirls over the patient's head. Different aspects of a patient's self become unified behind the scenes into a common approach. The patient may subsequently be faced with a kind of collusion against him or herself—albeit one sincerely thought to be for the patient's ultimate welfare.

I did not set out to mould my field research into a Goffmanian 'mortification of the self' perspective. Goffman analyses the 'abasements, degradations, humiliations, and profanations of self' experienced by the new patient in a total institution. The curtailments of self can occur even when the inmate is willing and the management has ideal concerns for his or her wellbeing. Mortifications are officially justified on a whole range of grounds—sanitation, responsibility for life, the necessity to look after a large number of people, the way things have to be now. In retrospect, however, my interpretation of my field research shows many similarities with Goffman's well known work. In severe body paralysis, the actual physical loss is the primary agent of mortification. But institutional imperatives and organisational logic also play a large part in the deconstitution of self. Although I acknowledge a strong affinity with Goffman's concept, I prefer to use the term transformation of self, and thereby avoid the emotional connotations associated with Goffman's term.

I have isolated five processes, which, I claim, propel the person towards becoming a patient: ascription of a diagnosis, a narrowed interactive area, uncertainty, isolation yet loss of privacy, and the control of information about the self by others. Although Goffman does not designate these processes in the same manner, the factors he isolates in his analysis of the moral career of the mental patient are similar in effect to those I have assigned transformative power.

In medical terms, 'patient' has a clear meaning. Definite relationships, appropriate behaviour and certain expectations are implicit in the word. A person becomes a patient at the moment a set of symptoms coincide with a medical syndrome. A patient is a medical entity: the subject of medical work.

For the individual, becoming a patient is more insidious. The experience of a paralysed body is new and confusing. Isolated in a narrowed, medically-oriented world, the paralysed person slowly comes to see him or herself as others do—as a patient.

7 Paralysed patient to person

This chapter deals in part with theoretical issues, of which Alfred Schutz's concept of multiple realities is the base. This discussion is necessary to establish the constitution of that finite province of meaning, which is the institutional reality, and to demonstrate the relationship of this province of meaning to the paramount reality of everyday life.

This sets the stage for a further transformation. Alternative ideas and meanings are mediated into the finite province of meaning of the patient by others. These ideas may modify, de-emphasize and subvert the person's previously dominant reality. Person, as an analytical label, marks that point at which an individual, having experienced trauma or disease, is able to incorporate physical deformities or great pain into a new and different, but for the person, ongoing self-definition of health.

Multiple realities

The world of daily life is an intersubjective world, existing before birth, and experienced and interpreted by others as well as ourselves as an organised world. In this world, men and women operate within the 'natural attitude' (Natanson, 1973:228). Within the natural attitude men and women unquestioningly accept their world; they take it for granted. Yet Schutz shows that other realities exist, each with its own special style of existence (Natanson, 1973:207). Schutz speaks of these realities as 'finite provinces of meaning'; as sets of experience which show a specific cognitive style and, with respect to this style, are not only consistent in themselves, but also compatible with one another (Natanson, 1973:230).

The world of everyday life is thus one finite province of meaning, among many others. But within the natural attitude the everyday world becomes *the* reality, the only way things can be, the paramount reality. We abandon our attitude towards any finite province of meaning by experiencing a specific shock, which compels us to break through the limits of this province of meaning and shift the accent of reality elsewhere (Natanson, 1973:231). Sudden, severe paralysis could constitute one such shock, which may compel the individual to pass from one finite province of meaning to another. A less dramatic yet perhaps more analytically convincing argument could be made to account for the relationship between the institutional province of meaning and the paramount reality of everyday life. The institutional province of meaning could be seen existing as a temporary enclave within the paramount reality of everyday life (Schutz and Luckman, 1973:127). The institutional reality becomes the finite province of meaning, disparate from the commonsense reality of everyday life, and possessing a distinctive cognitive style. All experiences within this small world are consistent in themselves and compatible with one another (Wagner, 1970:253). So long as the paralysed person partakes of the cognitive style of this particular province of meaning, it will be considered real; it will dominate his or her thinking, which will bestow upon it the accent of reality (Wagner, 1970:254).

Schutz claims that the multiple realities of non-pragmatic experiences are inferior to the paramount reality of everyday life, and in a sense remain dependent on it. When a person awakes from the world of dreams, for example, he or she returns to the more consistent and continuous world of everyday life.

Unlike the world of dreams, the institutional reality of the patient is a pragmatically constructed reality. But it too is ephemeral, and soon penetrated by the hard facts and realities of everyday life (Wagner, 1970:42). Yet as long as this reality remains, its style becomes dominant, and the demands and contingencies of the everyday world are suppressed. The realities of the everyday world assert their imposed relevances and subvert the institutional reality of the patient. This model is compatible with the analysis I wish to pursue here.

The paramount reality of everyday life experienced by an individual after disease or injury is, however, different from the paramount reality previously experienced by the person. Transformational processes have changed the meaning of the individual's experience. The new paramount reality of everyday life experienced by a paralysed person who sees him or herself as healthy, is an extension of Schutz's concept, but one that I believe would be compatible with his thesis.

The meaning province of the patient

When the person is transformed into a patient the definition of others may not be totally clear to him or her at this stage. But this does not alter its influence. Sooner or later the individual will come to see him or herself as a patient. This may happen early, in an institution, or later in the everyday world. But similar factors are instrumental in the transformation of meaning whenever and wherever it occurs.

Institutionalisation is inevitable in the early care of severely paralysed people. The enforced reconceptualisation of self, re-learning of formerly taken for granted skills, and reconstitution of relationships with others is undertaken in a medical world. The encompassing or 'total' (Goffman, 1968) character of the institution makes other realities in the everyday world seem remote and irrelevant. Encompassed within the reality of the institution (whether actual or conceptual) the individual comes to see him or herself as others do. The institutional reality becomes the person's dominant reality.

The enormity of Jim's paralysis and prolonged hospitalisation made his understanding of his condition difficult. He continued to think of his paralysis as a temporary disability. He 'knew' that as soon as he could stand out of bed his troubles would be over. Realisation that this was not to be came many months later when he was first stood up, with much human and mechanical support. This really upset him. 'It chipped away at what I thought I was.' For the first time Jim saw himself as a patient.

Because Jim was the youngest patient in the ward, he attracted a lot of attention from nurses and other staff. 'Nurses would drop in; there was lots of cheek—I really enjoyed having them around.' Jim's former orientation to sport and physical activities allowed him to gain some status in the rehabilitation programme because he was able to do some things a lot better than some of the other patients. 'The physiotherapist was quite excellent. She was able to set challenges I had some hope of meeting.'

But although Jim's new conception of himself was satisfactory to him in many ways, it was entirely related to the meaning province of a patient. The medical model of severe body paralysis had transformed the meaning of his experience. Neither the patient nor his significant others conceived of another reality. The everyday world, his former situation and relationships within it, had no meaning in the face of the dominant reality of the institutional world of the patient—which was now his world. Previously important others readjusted their conceptions of him in relation to the way he saw himself. Jim was firmly installed in the world of the patient. No other world had any meaning for him.

Bob, like Jim, was severely paralysed and spent a very long time in an institution. He too was not able to see a future outside the hospital. The hospital become his dominant reality. Although there were other young patients in this institution, the official policy was to separate the younger people from each other in order to leaven the predominantly geriatric work load for the staff. Bob, too, was able to develop social relationships with the nursing and domestic staff that were very satisfactory to him.

Frank's long hospitalisation was more of a time out from life. He did not see himself as a patient. He made few social contacts with others in the ward. He did not 'live' in the world of the patient, a world to which he had a legitimate passport. His eighteen months in an institution had no meaning. It was time that had to be passed before he resumed his life in the everyday world again. Not until Frank had been home and then returned to another hospital did he come to see himself as a patient; his experiences in the first institution became invested with meaning.

Although Maggie was severely affected by the polio virus and was totally dependent on mechanical devices for all her bodily functions for many months, she never lost sight of the fact that she would be going home. Unlike Bob and Jim she could always see another reality. But she too felt that the ward was the dominant reality for a long time, in fact long after she had gone home.

Michael, Phillip and Pam are traumatic paraplegics. Their physical disabilities are not as severe as the people I have just mentioned. Their stay in an institution was shorter, they were able to use wheelchairs early and gain some freedom denied to more severely paralysed people. All three continued to experience an outside social environment. Friendships with others in the everyday world continued throughout the rehabilitation period, and have remained constant. None of these people lost sight of the reality of everyday life. Yet each of them describes rehabilitation as a strongly influential time. Each sees, for a short time at least, the medical reality of paraplegia as the dominant reality.

Two worlds—alternative realities

The world of the patient is seen by the majority of my informants as distinct from the everyday world in which they formerly resided. Maggie describes the unreality of her first visits home, and the difficulties of re-establishing herself as a wife, mother, and indeed a woman, after her time as a patient. Jim saw his visits home as an afternoon's outing—no more than that. 'I didn't see myself settling back into it. I was going to live in the hospital. I was always pleased to get back to the hospital after a visit. I was secure there.'

Pam had very little disruption of her friendship relationships. Her friends and family were 'intellectually capable of accepting the disability. They never indicated to me that I was any different'. Pam was able to leave the hospital at quite an early stage in her rehabilitation programme to spend weekends at home. Yet even she says that she felt like 'Dr Jekyll and Mr Hyde' in her two worlds—the world of the patient and the world of everyday life.

The ward comes to have the security that was formerly associated with the home. Many patients speak of their fear of going out. Some look for excuses not to go out into the everyday world—to face the uncertainly and inconsistencies of a world that does not know or understand them. 'Going back into the world was like jumping a very high hurdle.' Jumping is impossible for the paralysed person. Reinserting oneself into everyday life may appear no less impossible.

In the patient's mind, the world of everyday life and the world of the patient may seem two distinct and incompatible realities. The everyday world relates to the former self, and as yet has no relevance for the present self. The world of the patient is consistently oriented around the new self, which as yet has not confronted his or her former social setting.

Yet the two realities may not be as distinct as they seem to the patient. The mandate of the staff to intrude beyond the physical confines of the hospital in order to plan a future for the patient has already been discussed in chapter 6. Although the patient is probably unaware of the dimensions of this knowledge, much information of his or her former social situation is carried into the world of the patient by professional information gatherers. This influences relationships in the institution.

On the other hand, the medical reality of the patient is mediated into the world of the everyday because of the institutional venue for the development of a new conception of self. An institution without walls—a tightly integrated medically-oriented reality, may persist in the patient's mind and thus influence his or her interactions with others long after the patient has left the institution.

Becoming a person again does not necessarily coincide with discharge from the institution. It may occur totally within the institution, or it may occur long after the patient has left this temporarily dominant province of meaning.

So the world of the patient and the everyday world are in fact thoroughly interwoven. The outside world permeates the hospital; the hospital flows into the outside world. But this is not the way the majority of my informants perceived these alternative realities. How does the individual escape the imposed relevances of the institution? Is there a way out?

Will power

Will power is an issue that is raised time and time again by staff, patients and others as the agent of transformation from patient to person. Popular understandings attribute great potential to the human will. The triumph of the human spirit over an appalling and devastating situation is the theme of much literature (Sontag, 1979) and mass media coverage. 'If you believe in yourself you will come through whatever. Take hold of yourself: life is in the palm of your hands.' 'With an accident like this you would have to be a fool not to come out a better person.' 'There is no good reason for losing your independence except your own will power.' These statements were made to me by paraplegics. But many professional people, trained in the 'science of medicine', have denied the logic of their training by attributing the progress of paralysed people to such a force (Balint, 1957:216).

Undoubtedly the power of the human will must play a part in the return to health of people who are severely paralysed. But will power is not a personal property the individual brings preformed to the rehabilitative task. To focus on this is to do a grave disservice to many such people who for a whole variety of physical, structural, situational, social or economic reasons may be less able to resume a satisfactory way of life. The individual will is powerless by itself. the will must be given the social and structural room to move. Any of these factors can assist or prevent the human will from attaining its goal.

Guts, motivation, moral fibre, strength of character—these

attributes are too often raised to be ignored. But attributing rehabilitative potential to such psychological factors puts a heavy load on the individual. These factors must be given the space to operate by wider factors not wholly contained within the individual's mind. Social and structural issues impose on the efforts of the individual's mind and influence the ability of the will to operate. The mediating agents may be social not psychological; the limitations may be structural not moral.

Mediators

Social mediators introduce inconsistent and divergent ideas to challenge the dominance of the medical reality. These ideas are resources which enable the patient to stand apart from the medical reality, to reflect on it and to see it in relation to everyday life (Kapferer, 1979). Over time, the inconsistent ideas allow the patient the conceptual room to reorder and rearrange his or her ideas in reference to another reality, that of the everyday world to which he or she has related, and may again relate.

The ideas that penetrate the omnipotence of the patient's world may appear trivial and of small consequence. But they enable the patient to hold off the institutional reality for a while and reflect on the possibility of an alternative point of view. These ideas have no deterministic quality in their own right. They may be picked up differentially by a patient because they relate to an experience or an idea that has relevance and meaning for him or her, either retrospectively or in relation to a future projection.

Staff as mediators

Anselm Strauss et al define their concept of 'sentimental work' as work done specifically with regard to the responses of the person or persons worked with, and done in the service of the main line of work. This type of work amounts to necessary, but institutionally unaccountable work, such as reassuring a child while a doctor performs a painful procedure, or of comforting an anxious cancer sufferer while radiotherapy treatment proceeds.

In a spinal injuries or diseases unit, however, this type of staff mediation is seen as integral to medical work. It is a distinctive characteristic of the work done in such institutions, and as such is organisationally accounted for. But the personal nature of this type of interaction makes it potentially problematic for all concerned.

For both Bob and Jim, this type of sentimental work served its avowed purpose of making these men feel less object-like—of personalising the treatment programme to make it easier for the staff to pursue. The unintended, but always possible, consequence of this type of work is that by the provision of areas of satisfactory interaction within the institutional context, the world of the patient is deepened and expanded to the detriment of the outside world.

A physiotherapist may spend many hours a day with a paralysed patient. A physiotherapist works on a 9–5 basis. She or he is not under the same type of organisational control as the nursing staff, and has more autonomy in treatment allocation and procedures.

Both Bob and Jim developed strong and important relationships with women physiotherapists during their institutional stay. Both claim that the physiotherapists treated them like equals; that they saw them as allies against the regular staff. The physiotherapist was able to set small challenges that the patient had some hope of attaining. Institutionally legitimated sentimental work can very easily turn into a more serious personal relationship in this context. While this type of interaction may be extremely important and beneficial for the patient, it may also serve to push the individual even further into the world of the patient, and further distance him or her from the everyday world.

The patient looks more and more to the achievement of 'patient goals' for satisfaction. The outside world becomes more and more remote. 'I did not want to go back to being a husband or a father. I was secure where I was. I became a bit of a king. I was the youngest in the ward. Nurses would drop in. I had a little 'fridge with beer. Everything outside became unreal. I didn't want to go back to that.'

Sentimental work succeeded in making the patient less object-like, in personalising the organisational routines. But the precarious nature of the alternative realities in such a context had the unintended consequence of orienting the individual even more to the world of the patient, and away from the reality of everyday life.

I do not wish to emphasise this detrimental effect of sentimental work to the exclusion of the more positive effects. Unlike Strauss et al, who see this work as exclusively promoting the smooth execution of organisational work, I see these interactions frequently working against the dominance of the insitutional order. Staff have professional ideologies, but they also bring to their work understandings selected from their total social experience. In another work, Strauss suggests that nursing aides, usually untrained practical nurses, play an important role in interaction with patients in a psychiatric institution (1963:158). Aides are more likely to be the recipients of patients' conversations and confidences because of their frequent and intimate contact with the patient. Aides guide themselves by many commonsense maxims. They interact with the patient in less professionalised, non-medical terms, and are thus privy to a different level of problems, which might not be raised with other more professional staff.

Trips to football games, shopping centres and movies with the staff are occasions for a flood of new meanings to enter the patient's understanding of him or herself. Away from the institutional context, yet with the security of expert help for practical problems, both former assumptions and institutional wisdom are modified as the individual moves toward a new self-understanding.

Bob, like Jim, was able to develop important interrelationships with members of the staff of the institution. 'One nurse was really incredible...She really got me alive. She introduced me to all sorts of new ideas. I could really have an intellectual conversation with her.' The woman Bob subsequently married was on the staff of the institution also. She was very important in subverting the reality of the institution for Bob. The introduction of ideas from the everyday world into Bob's world enabled him to shore up this reality for a time and reflect on the possibility of an alternative reality. She was able to introduce ideas and possibilities that Bob could gradually weave into an emerging new self.

Although he still lives within an institution, a close relationship with a former staff member has also been important for Frank's transformation from patient to person. The transformation is not yet complete, but the goal is in sight. Since he met his friend three years ago, Frank has 'got himself sorted out'. 'We talk about all sorts of things. She has meant a lot to me.' The close relationship and frequent contact with a friend in the outside world has subverted the reality of the institution for Frank. 'Now I know what the problem is, and I know what has to be done. I don't let anyone get on top of me. But it has not always been so.' Frank is now able to see his very real physical limitations in terms of the everyday world. He sees himself as a person, and although still living in an institution, is able to contemplate a time when he will live outside it. His physical disabilities take on the nature of practical problems that can be overcome, in contrast to their former status as the focus of a tightly intermeshed, medically-oriented reality.

Phillip also found that interaction with the younger staff was important in assessing his potential for interaction in the everyday world once he left the institution. 'I often asked the younger nurses what they would think of developing a friendship with a person in a wheelchair. This way you could get an idea of how they, as people in the outside world, would react to someone like you.'

Patients as mediators

Some patients, however, claim that the staff can do no more than the regular work of the institution. The staff, they consider, are not capable of understanding the patient as anything more than the object of medical work. The staff are incapable of conceiving what the physical disabilities mean to the specific individual. 'What would they know? They're not in the same position. They can walk. Expert knowledge is very different from experience knowledge.'

Michael, in particular, held this opinion very strongly. During his stay in the institution he organised a 'sub-culture' of patients who were able to distance themselves from the professional assumptions of the organisation. 'The only person who can teach a paraplegic what to do is another paraplegic. The only person who can teach a quadriplegic is another quadriplegic.' 'We did what we wanted. They were looking after their interests and we were looking after ours.'

Information passed between patients, although mostly about practical problems or the difficulties encountered on visits home, enabled other patients to project themselves into similar situations. This could lead to the rehabilitation programme within the institution being more profitably utilised, because the patient was able to relate this work to a goal outside the hospital. Patients closer to discharge from the institution, or old paraplegics or quadriplegics coming back are particularly helpful in discussing sexual possibilities and other more intimate aspects of personal relationships. Although these issues are sometimes discussed with the patient by the staff, the abstract nature of such discussion provides little understanding to the patient of the actual meaning of such a loss for him or her.

The assumptions of the 'patient sub-culture' within the institution described by Michael may, in fact, have been more encompassing for some patients than the assumptions of the staff. 'We made patients accept their problem. You had two choices—either accept and enjoy it, or get out of the chair and walk out of the hospital and pretend there is nothing wrong with you. We didn't accept "no" for an answer. And you couldn't say, "Oh yes, but it's easier for you". We used to give the patients a hard time.'

Patients may be strongly critical of what they see as another patient's refusal to 'make the most of it'. The moral implication of 'if I can do it so can you' often ignores the fact that a different set of physical problems may exist, and certainly a whole variety of less amenable social, economic or occupational arrangements may apply. Patients may introduce positive ideas to other patients. But by challenging the medically-constructed reality, other patients can set themselves up as being more expert than the medical experts, and thus construct for some patients an even more formidable reality.

The tuberculosis hospital studied by Roth, whilst an inmate himself, bears many similarities to a spinal unit (1963). Patients have varying degrees of the same injury and receive similar treatment. All are mentally intact, and expect to spend a long time in the institution. Such common problems can provoke a solidarity of patient interests, and a perception of themselves as the experts on treatment and institutional living.

Apart from the example of patient solidarity told me by Michael, my investigations suggest that this probably seldom happens. Age, sex, social class, varying stages of rehabilitation, the continual admission and discharge of patients cut across factors that could lead to solidarity. The sense of being more expert than the 'experts' is certainly often expressed, though while the patient remains in the institution, this understanding is unlikely to lead to patient solidarity.

Others as mediators

There is no doubt that, initially at least, the transformation from patient to person was more smoothly executed by those people who had well developed social relationships before their injury.

Elements of these relationships had to be rearranged and reordered. Yet a strong and continuous bond stretched through the institutional reality and enabled the re-establishment of an ongoing, although transformed healthy self. Because these people never lost sight of the reality of everyday life, they never became submerged in the institutional reality. They were able to use the facilities of the rehabilitation unit in a more practical sense. The mediators of their conceptual transformation were participating members of the everyday world—people who had contributed to the individual's previous conception of self, and people who were in the position to do so again by accomodating the change.

Michael, Phillip and Pam were in this position. Each of them was well supported by family and friends. Early weekend leave from the ward allowed these important relationships to proceed, predominantly in the everyday world. Pam's previous involvement in singing was an important mediator for her. Instead of performing in a forthcoming light opera production, she was immediately put in charge of costuming and makeup. This involvement required a weekly outing from the rehabilitation unit. The nature of her participation in this activity had certainly changed, but her involvement with others from her former self-conception was continuous with her new self-conception. Both Pam and her significant others were able to rearrange a new and ongoing conception of self, with a sense of history and continuity.

Phillip, like Pam, had ongoing support from family, friends and girlfriend. These people were able to reassure Phillip that there was a place for him in the outside world, both conceptually and actually. He, like Michael and Pam, was able to use the rehabilitation unit more as a practical, problem-solving agency.

Other patients, particularly, it seems from my observations young men, have more difficulty. Many men in their late teenage years have left their natal home but have not yet formed a close set of alternative people to mediate their reintegration into the everyday world. In a broad sense, primary socialisation is a person's evolution from dependence to independence through the stages of infancy, childhood, adolescence and young adulthood. Having so recently claimed their independence from their family, the necessity to re-enter the relationship on such dependent terms may be severely detrimental to the development of a new conception of self.

My field observations led me to focus mainly on the staff and other patients as mediators. Both groups of people are within the institution, a seeming contradiction to my theme. Yet the fact that these people are located within the institution may increase the effectiveness of the everyday ideas they unwittingly disseminate within the patient's world.

The intermeshed ideas of the finite province of meaning dominate a patient's thoughts for a time. But patients arrive, go home, are discharged, and return in a continuous stream. Patients are not an homogeneous group. Someone is always becoming a patient, as another patient is returning to health.

Outsiders can look on the objective facts of the patient's condition from another perspective. They do not share the patient's relationship to the framework of ideas within the institution. The outsider is able to assess the standards prevailing within the finite province of meaning in relation to a system of relevances current in the everyday world. Members of an outgroup do not hold the ways of life in the ingroup as self-evident truths (Wagner, 1970:85). Outsider others are undoubtedly in a good position to subvert the finite province of meaning for the patient. Yet the ideas of others can also be severely detrimental to the transformation of a patient to a person, an issue to be discussed in the next chapter.

My analysis has focussed on the human mediating agents of transformation. But mediation is achieved not only in face to face situations. Diverse ideas from many sources, past, present and future, reintroduce the everyday into the patient's narrowed world. These ideas allow the patient to hold off the institutional reality, and reflect on the possibility of alternative meanings. A transformation of meaning for the patient occurs when the relevances and typifications of the institutional reality are subverted, and the person can reconstruct a new self in relation to the relevances and typifications of the everyday world.

8 Barriers to transformation

In the preceding chapter I discussed the introduction of divergent ideas into the patient's world by mediators both within and outside this province of meaning. 'Others' made it possible for the patient to become a person. Although discursive ideas came from many and diverse sources, the focus of this chapter was on ideas generated through language and in face to face situations.

This analysis followed symbolic interactionist theory. Basic to this perspective is the idea that the self is established, maintained and altered through communication. Most investigators have emphasised language as the crucial element in communication. Certainly verbal discourse has been an important issue in the analysis of the negation and reconstruction of the self pursued in chapters 6 and 7.

But language is not the only dimension of exchange in interaction. The physical appearance of the people involved may be equally important to the nature of the interaction that can develop. As previously mentioned, I possess my body in a much more thoroughgoing and immediate sense than I can possess other objects. It is this intimacy of possession that is the source of such devastation to the severely disabled person. Major alterations to the appearance and functioning of the body challenge the intimacy of this relationship and can constitute a disembodiment. Suddenly the self has been stripped from its corporeal moorings. The person is no longer what he or she understands him or herself to be.

A person develops an awareness of his or her body by the experience of living in that body. However, because the body in which the person lives is visible to others, it is the object of social attention and public appraisal. Social interactions provide the person with critical data for knowledge of his or her body.

The exterior of the body is the medium by which the individual is represented in public. The self is continuously constituted in face to face interaction. Most people have a large repertoire of techniques to change their appearance to an image they wish to present to others.

The social aspects of the body do not end with the flesh and bones of the human form, 'For the apparel oft proclaims the man', as Polonius says in *Hamlet*. Discernment, taste and savoir faire are expressed by dress; class position is made manifest by the cut, texture and colour of dress, suit and jacket. Particular dress is associated with certain types of social events. 'Black tie' involves rather more garments than the term implies, yet 'black tie' would be considered overdressing for a barbecue. Academic gowns and hoods are ceremonial vestiges of past eras, yet are still worn by members of high table at antipodean universities. The hostess who advises her guests not to dress for dinner would be horrified if they obeyed her instructions.

Clothing is much more than a protective covering for the body. Buttoning the collar on men's shirts, rolling up the sleeves, letting the shirt hang outside the trousers are all stylistic features, which in a particular social context will convey precise social messages (Polhemus, 1978:ch.8). Fashion trends in clothing, dress codes of both conformity and rebellion, and personal choices and styles of dress are social products whereby the individual expresses his or her identity and social place.

Even those people who claim indifference to the tools of appearance manipulation cannot escape their influence. Whoever eschews the latest cut in trousers or fashion in hair design, or neglects to wash or groom themselves still presents a powerful body image for public scrutiny. We have the power to effect considerable control over the way we appear to others.

The newly-disabled person presents a visual image to the world that bears little resemblance to the way the person sees him or herself. Moreover, people react to the person on the basis of this external image. Others alienate the person from his or her inner awareness of self, yet the reactions of others are essential to complete the self-image of the person, an image that the person him or herself can only partially complete (Mead, 1934).

Unlike language, which is discursive in nature, the physical appearance of a person is non-discursive, or presentational in character (Kapferer, 1979). It is directly given to the other. The appearance of a visibly disabled person immediately provokes cultural understandings and assumptions about his or her nature in the minds of others. Perception and assumptions are fused into one (Wagner, 1970:31). As Schutz says, by the visual perception of another's body and its movements, a system of well ordered indications of his psychological life and his experience is constituted (quoted in Wagner, 1970:164).

The presentational nature of physical appearance can establish processes that act against the reconstruction of a person from a patient in interaction in the everyday world. The physical appearance of the visibly disabled person is presented to others as is, as an undifferentiated whole, as an unquestionable reality. Perception provokes assumptions. The perception by others of the physical appearance of the visibly disabled may deny the person his or her full transformative potential. A limited transformation may occur. The person's self-conception may retain elements of patienthood because of the continued understandings of others, based on the way he or she is seen by them. Others interact with the person in terms of assumptions based on physical appearance. Others may sustain the person as a patient, preventing full conceptional transformation as a healthy person again.

Gregory Stone (1962) works strictly in the mode of G. H. Mead as expressed in symbolic interactionist theory. Nevertheless he is critical of the neglect of the non-verbal dimension of interaction by many writers in this perspective. Stone seeks to widen the boundaries of symbolic interactionism by including a consideration of the appearance of the participants in interaction on equal terms with the verbal communication between them. Goffman (1959, 1971) has also considered physical appearance in many of his analyses.

For Mead, meaning in social transactions is guaranteed by role-taking, by placing oneself in the attitude of the other. This ensures that one's own response will be more, rather than less, coincident with the response of the other, since the other's incipient actions have become incorporated in the actions of the one producing the symbol (Mead, 1934:254). Stone considers that confluence of meaning in interaction is better conceptualised by the term 'identification' than by Mead's 'role-taking'. The two processes—identification of and identification with—are facilitated by appearance. 'Appearance sets the stage for, permits, sustains and delimits the possibilities of discourse by underwriting the possibilities of meaningful discussion' (Stone, 1962:90). A dialectic interrelationship of appearance and discourse characterises all interaction. Stone's insights are relevant for all interaction but they are particularly relevant for the issues addressed here. Constant or chronic pain may also affect a person's self-concept and interaction with others, yet is invisible—a useful corrective to the emphasis on visible appearance pursued in this chapter (Kotarba, 1977).

Very definite changes in the external appearance of a person accompany severe body paralysis. A high-level quadriplegic has very little neck movement. His or her upper extremities hang heavily from the shoulders; the hands lie curled inwards at the wrists. Before long the paralysis of the muscles of the trunk produce a 'pot-bellied' appearance with a pronounced shortening of the seated body. Wasting of the leg muscles causes a 'stick-legged' appearance of the lower extremities. After intensive rehabilitation, a paraplegic is likely to have well developed shoulders and arms. Depending on the level of the injury, he or she too may develop the 'pot-bellied' appearance caused by paralysis or weakness of the abdominal muscles.

The necessity for mechanical aids increases the visibility of these physical disabilities. A wheelchair is an unequivocal symbol of permanent physical loss. Some less disabled paraplegics are able to walk with a large amount of orthopedic gear, although even these people spend the majority of their time in a wheelchair.

All paralysed people are limited in the ways they can create and control their appearance. High-level quadriplegics can't raise their arms to do their hair or clean their teeth. They are not able to dress themselves, or to rearrange or adjust aspects of their appearance that displease them. These limitations are severe in quadriplegics. But even paraplegics are faced with severe curtailment of the usual ways of controlling one's appearance.

For men, a plastic, see-through urinary drainage bag is permanently strapped to the ankle. Long trousers must be worn to cover this external plumbing apparatus. The difficulty in pulling trousers on over paralysed legs, together with the perennial risk of pressure sores from sitting on hard or creased fabric, means that soft, pull-on trousers of the 'track-suit' variety become characteristic dress for paralysed people. Paralysed feet are vulnerable to chilblains, sunburn and physical trauma because the paralysed person is no longer able to feel when this damage is occurring. Many paralysed people wear large wool boots such as 'Ug Boots' to minimise this type of damage.

As well as these static elements of appearance, non-verbal communication is also facilitated in everyday life by subtle, yet critical expressions such as gestures, body contact, posture and facial expression (Polhemus, 1978). These elements are largely taken for granted in social interaction. The face is the most important area for non-verbal expression (Argyle, 1975:211). Mercifully this avenue of communication is available to all paralysed people. A paraplegic man, discussing his own potential in comparison to a quadriplegic said, 'There would be nothing worse than being a complete quadriplegic. You have nothing wrong with your brain...but your whole body is tied up. All you are is a head—a head that just sits there'. Denied the use of the hands, body and feet in communication, a quadriplegic person soon comes to realise the importance of facial expression in interaction.

But bodily movements, posture, spatial position and bodily contact are also important components of non-verbal communication. The importance of these factors in underpinning interaction is taken for granted until the physical means of their expression is no longer possible. Frank expresses his sadness that he has never been able to pick up and cuddle his then baby, now early teenage, daughter. Phillip, a young paraplegic, comparing himself to a quadriplegic said, 'It would really depress me if I couldn't hug someone'.

More subtle, yet no less important, expressive modes of communication may also be lost. In non-paralysed people messages from the body surface are received by the brain, which in turn guides body movements. Contact with the body stimulates an awareness of touch, pressure, warmth, cold, pain (Argyle, 1975: 286). Not only is the sensory apprehension of these aspects of bodily contact lost, but the physical ability to respond appropiately no longer exists.

Posture, stance, the physical orientation of the body in space can no longer be controlled by the individual to his or her own satisfaction, but are entirely determined by the extent of the disability and mechanical aids.

Most of the paralysed people to whom I have spoken have strongly emphasised the need to orient themselves to the everyday world. Davis calls this 'normalisation', a favoured strategy since our society places such store in 'the normal', 'the healthy' and 'the physically attractive' (Davis, 1963:157). Implementation is, of course, easier for Michael, Phillip and Pam than it is for Frank.

Physical appearance was always an important issue for Michael. 'It is very important to me not to look like a cripple. I am in a chair, but I don't want to look like a cripple. I don't want stuff around me that looks as though it has been especially made for me. I want things to look as normal and everyday as possible.'

Although a barber regularly visits the institution where Frank lives, he prefers to arrange to go to a barber outside the hospital. Although this involves a considerable amount of organisation, he prefers to do it because 'it is important to do things like everyone else.'

Phillip could, with a lot of effort, walk with the aid of orthopedic support but the security of a wheelchair allows him to create and control other aspects of his appearance. 'Your hands are free. You look more natural in a chair.'

Pam's loss of waistline, due to abdominal muscle paralysis, still concerns her. Dresses no longer suit her. She says it took a long time before she could find clothing that satisfied both her understanding of herself and her altered physical state. She describes her fears on receiving an invitation to a wedding. 'How will I ever be able to go?' The necessity of controlling the nature of interaction in such a large, variable and unknown setting is fraught with anxiety. 'You have to rethink yourself into every possibility of formerly taken for granted situations.'

Although paralysed people see themselves as physically different, these people strongly resist and reject the imputation of others that they are socially different. 'After all it's a broken back, not a broken mind. You're still a person. You may be disabled, but your brain hasn't gone. But unfortunately some people do assume that your personality has changed.' A joking conversation between two men, both high-level quadriplegics in wheelchairs, illustrates a modest attempt to challenge the popular meaning of 'normal'. A group of young women, presumably visiting nurses, entered the ward: 'Who are they?' 'Don't know'. 'Are they walking?' 'Must be peculiar. Only peculiar people use feet not wheels!'

Able-bodied people find it impossible to imagine themselves paralysed. Because we are a body and because we also have bodies, we cannot contemplate not being a body, or having a body at our disposal. To try to understand the sensory, functional and conceptual losses that the individual is experiencing, while confronted by his or her vivid corporeal presence is too perverse for most people to contemplate. How can an able-bodied person imagine how it feels not to feel?

Michael classifies able-bodied people in three ways—'Those who accept you and treat you like a person; those people who would rather ignore you than include you, or else become overly sympathetic, and a third group who can't face the fact that you are a person, that you feel like them and have the same needs and desires.' All of the people I spoke with suggested similar impediments to interaction.

Pam suggests that the sympathy of many people can overwhelm the possibilities of more satisfactory interaction. As a participant observer, I was not immune from this danger myself. On an outing to a suburban shopping centre, we stopped to eat lunch. Bill, a high-level quadriplegic, was eating his lunch with extreme difficulty. I heard him say that he wished that he had remembered to bring a fork. Overcome with sympathy for him, I rushed to a nearby shop to get a fork. It was not until I had handed the fork to him that I realised that not only could he not reach out to take it from me, but manipulation of food into his mouth with it would be impossible. When he had said 'fork', he had meant an extensive arm splint with an attachment for a specially adapted fork. Interaction with Bill was on my terms. When the interaction ended in disaster, I was able to indulge my embarrassment by avoiding him for the rest of the day. My thoughtless sympathy further reinforced for Bill his 'not normal' state.

On the same trip to the shopping centre, I accompanied Jean, an older paraplegic woman, to look at television sets. Although there were no other customers in the department, the salesman studiously ignored us. When I eventually demanded that he attend to Jean, he insisted on talking to me despite my continual efforts to redirect the conversation. Jean's quick decision to buy an expensive, remote-controlled, coloured television provoked visible uneasiness in the salesman. Balancing the reality of a 600 dollar sale with assumptions of social deviancy, if not frank mental deficiency, was a precarious affair. The suggestion that the set be delivered to the hospital tomorrow rather than taken straight away allowed the salesman to conclude the transaction without too much at stake.

Maggie had discussed with me that while older people became cautious and over-polite in relating to her, young children stared at her and often asked direct questions. I could see by Ann's uneasiness at the approach of a small child at the shopping centre that she had also experienced the frankness of children's curiosity. On this occasion, however, the child lent both elbows on the arms of Ann's chair, and quite oblivious to Ann's disability or her presence in a wheelchair, proceeded to discuss with

Ann her father's imminent birthday and the difficulty in choosing a present for him.

Bob's own son, born after his father was paralysed from poliomyelitis, spent several of his adolescent years pretending that he didn't know his father. He would not allow his father to come to his school: in public he insisted on walking far ahead or far behind Bob's wheelchair.

The assumptions of others can cause a 'stickiness of interactional flow', (Davis, 1964:120). The visibility of the disability can seriously challenge the framework of normative rules and assumptions in which sociability usually develops. The effort to avoid taboo words and topics puts great strain on the free flow of conversation (Goffman, 1961:47). To be sensitive to the way the disabled person wishes to see him or herself without letting sympathy for his or her physical state engulf the interaction is difficult. Patronising and condescending remarks—'How nice you have something to do', or 'How strange that someone so pretty should be in a wheelchair'—serve to reinforce the limited parameters of the patient's world and reaffirm how far he or she has yet to move to gain relevance in the larger everyday world.

Pam is often asked to talk at public meetings about paraplegia. Having made preliminary arrangements on the telephone about a particular speaking engagement, Pam asks, 'What is the access to your building like because I am in a wheelchair?' On many occasions, the speaker on the other end of the telephone line has said, 'My golly, you don't *sound* as though you are in a wheelchair!' 'They have their set ideas that I sound "normal." When I say that I am in a wheelchair, their conception of me is confused.'

Yet sometimes the assumptions of paralysed people about themselves are more serious deterrents to interactional flow than the ideas of others. The paralysed person will not be free of the popular assumptions towards the handicapped, since he or she was once a participating member of the everyday world. Frank has developed a very important relationship with a woman, a former nurse in the institution where he now lives. 'She has even gone as far as offering me a ticket out of here. (I assume this to mean marriage or a permanent domestic relationship). But it would be against my nature. I have always felt that if I couldn't put my share into something, I wouldn't do it at all.'

Other paralysed people have told me that they can see, in retrospect, that it was their own understandings of themselves at a particular time or in a certain context that were formidable barriers to transformation. The responses of oneself to one's own appearance and body state can be as important to the nature of the interaction that can develop as the meaning of the appearance of disabled people to others.

The interactional problems encountered by a person with a visible disability are of the same type that we all encounter from time to time in our social lives. In our daily lives we all display signs that allow others to identify us and to make assumptions about us. In turn, we pick up clues from the clothing, posture, gait, gestures and mannerisms of the people we meet in order to provide us with information about those parts of their lives that are less visible to us. It is easy to imagine that we know a lot more about a person from these presentational clues than is actually the case. Yet no matter how tentative the actual connection between the exterior characteristics of a person and his or her inner nature, the effect of such evaluations is immense. Although we may use diverse strategies to deflect the assumptions of others or protect ourselves from scrutiny, ultimately even these devices may become the source of evidence for further assumptions about us. An old person dressing in fashions intended for a younger person, or a working-class person wearing a Bermuda yachting jacket at the weekend may not only fail to achieve their intended goal, but may also provide others with further evidence of their personality.

Clearly gender, age and race are powerful visual interactive agents. Such strong bodily presentations dominate the nature of the interaction that can take place. The external image of an older Italian woman, for example, stimulates a flood of generalities to crowd the observer's mind. Such generalities may bear little or no relation to the actual person, yet will become the basis upon which the observer relates or chooses to ignore that person. The gender, age and racial aspects of the person's bodily appearance become detached from her essential identity and from her biographical and social past from which her identity arose. She may be given no opportunity to refute or dispute the assumptions with which she has been invested since any possibility of discourse may be aborted on the basis of her appearance.

Such exclusions and role constrictions are common responses of people to the appearance of others, yet seldom can the criteria for such actions be openly discussed. Not to be asked to dance, not to be asked to join the club—what does this mean? Such issues can seldom be explored since their meaning is hidden under layers of 'civilised' behaviour, and thus defies examination. But although such actions may elude logical analysis, this in no way diminishes their effectiveness. We all have bodies, and we all have eyes to perceive the bodies of others. Such observations are inevitable; no matter how unjust, no matter how irrelevant, such judgements are essential mechanisms of social life.

Although the assumptions of others may sometimes preclude all possibility of discourse, most often the assumptions of others about us become obvious in subsequent interaction. Sometimes the ideas others have about us fit with the understandings we have of ourselves. Sometimes they do not. Most people have a wide range of strategies to redress the discrepancy between the way others see them and the way they see themselves or to insulate themselves from the displeasing assumptions of others. Sometime a mild conversational corrective will suffice, other times a more confrontational strategy may be required. A resolution to avoid drinking in the same bar, or to change a tutorial group may be enough to hold off the discrepant ideas, but a more serious decision to avoid the person altogether may be needed to alleviate the influence of the identity-threatening assumptions of others.

Such interactional dilemmas are shared by us all. We all make judgements about people on the basis of their appearance; we have all experienced the distress of discrepant assumptions of others about us. We have all felt excluded, we have all felt constrained by a set of stereotypic ideas indiscriminately applied to us in social situations. But the bodies of people with visible disabilities are different, they are conspicuous in social contexts. Such people have fewer means of protecting themselves from the scrutiny of others, and far less expressive and interactional resources to redress the identity-denying components of social intercourse. An examination of the breakdown of the framework of normative rules and assumptions that usually guide social interaction, through the minds of permanently and visibly disabled people, can illuminate important but usually taken for granted aspects of all social interaction.

Social barriers to transformation are omnipresent and oppressive. I have discussed at length the relevance of appearance in the reconstitution of a healthy self. But many other barriers may prevent transformation. A whole variety of structural, economic and physical factors may impede the reconstruction of self. The patient may be prevented from total transformation by elements located entirely outside him or herself and his or her particular social context. The range of choices may seem large, but in fact is severely circumscribed by social structural forces. Certain behaviour is permitted within a social context; other behaviour implicitly outlawed. Many ways in which a person may wish to reconstitute him or her self may be socially inappropriate. Gender assumptions may impede successful reconstitution of the self, as may many dominant ideas about sexuality and sexual practices. These issues will be discussed further in chapter 9. Class inequalities are more profoundly experienced by people whose opportunities are already curtailed by physical loss.

At a personal level, financial considerations are important elements in the mediation of a patient to a person. Some traumatic injuries attract large amounts of compensation. Diving accidents and poliomyelitis receive nothing; in fact the patient is often liable for huge bills for hospitalisation. There is no doubt that a patient's financial resources affect his or her ability to reorganise everyday life in practical terms, and thus influence the reconception of self.

The political determination of architectural, occupational, educational and consumer priorities is unresponsive to the needs of the majority of the population. The disabled may be effectively disenfranchised by these instrumentalities. Structural barricades in the form of architectural obstructions, legislative impediments and occupational deterrents act silently but surely against the total transformation of a patient to a healthy person again. Toilets without provision for wheelchair users, narrow supermarket checkouts, the camber on a footpath, and automatic lift doors which close too quickly are common features of the everyday world. But each of these can seem an insurmountable barrier to the reconstruction of a healthy self.

Furthermore, physical disability or pain may be so severe that the person is unable to think of him or herself as anything but a patient. They may not be able to reject the disease status completely. Some elements of the disease may be retained; the individual may feel he or she is not completely cured. A limited transformation has occurred. The patient has been transformed into a person, but a person with a disease. As a person, the individual interacts with others in the everyday world, but relations are modified by others' understanding of the person's restricted conception of him or herself. The understandings that others adopt towards the person can sustain the person as a patient, and prevent his or her complete conceptual transformation as a healthy person.

9 What is health after disease or trauma?

Despite these limitations, many people are able to make the transformation from patient to person. A complete transformational rearrangement of meaning occurs when a person, having experienced trauma or disease, is able to incorporate physical disabilities, deformities, or large amounts of pain into a new and different, but for the person ongoing self-definition of health.

These disturbances of bodily appearance, function and perception are quite inconsistent with the criteria the individual would previously have used to evaluate his or her health. Such physical disabilities and bodily malfunctions are quite at variance with popular cultural understandings of health. Yet the individual is able to accommodate such inconsistencies. The person is able to reconceptualise these elements into his or her own understanding of health, and reorder the understandings of others and the manner in which they interact. The person sees him or herself as healthy.

But the physical disabilities persist. I do not wish to trivialise the very real handicaps these present to paralysed people. I suggest, though, that now the physical loss is seen as just that—a handicap, a hindrance to the pursuance of everyday life, but not as an impossible barricade against the conception of a healthy self.

Structured systems of body behaviour vary from society to society, but must be learned by people if they are to interact successfully with other people in that society (Birdwhistell, 1972). Awkward or inappropriate body behaviour provokes the attention of others in ways which may be very detrimental to future interaction.

The difference between sex and gender is not mere pedantics; it is a critical distinction. Sex refers to the basic anatomical and physiological differences between males and females, the genetically determined and largely universal distinctions between men and women. Gender, on the other hand, refers to the culturally specific patterns of behaviour that are attached to the sexes. Masculinity and femininity are socially determined, and are therefore highly variable, manifestations of gender (Oakley, 1972).

Gender categories would not 'stick' however, no matter how formidably they are applied, unless such distinctions were underwritten by more substantial structures. In most societies, males have more power and more authority than women, and moreover, they have power over women. Men and women are thus not merely different, but more significantly, they relate together within a structure of subordination and domination called patriachy (Bilton et al., 1981:323). Even before the baby boy is dressed in blue and the baby girl in pink, gender-specific expectations and assumptions crowd into the developing infant's world. Many studies provide convincing evidence that the educational system reinforces gender divisions rather than challenging them (Bilton et al., 1981:ch.7). As if the family and the school were not influential enough, adolescent peer groups, the mass media, and language further cement masculine and feminine behaviour into socially prescribed categories.

What does gender mean for the person with a disability? What impact do such social categories have on the transformation of a patient into a healthy person again? Does 'masculinity' impede or facilitate the social integration of a man with a disability? Are disabled women further handicapped by the prescriptive nature of 'femininity'? If society's powerful gender-specific elements were influential in the person's previous conception of self, can that person transcend his or her body in order to form a satisfactory new self-concept of health?

Quadriplegia and paraplegia have sexual implications. Sexuality can often involve vulnerability and uncertainty about one's body appearance and performance. Insecurities about the way others see us and a fear of rejection by those people we most wish to impress are anxieties we have all experienced. We all develop complex protective mechanisms to defend ourselves from more physical and emotional exposure than we feel able to deal with. Nevertheless, sexual relationships inevitably involve taking emotional risks, and learning to deal with the consequences. Such risk taking can enhance excitement and be an important stimulus for arousal and pleasurable sexual activity in able-bodied people.

Sexuality for the man or woman with a disability, on the other hand, can take on formidable dimensions. The trauma or the disease has alienated the person from his or her body. Not only is the body estranged from the self but the body is no longer capable of feeling or reacting to stimuli in the same way. Previous understandings about the body, its attractiveness to others and preferred modes of sexual activity, are no longer relevant. The body as a sexual entity has been negated. This loss may be the most significant barrier to successful reconstitution of a healthy self. The disabled man or woman has built up a sexual identity of him or herself in the able-bodied world. Intimate relationships with others are valuable sources of body knowledge. Memories of these important identity-creating relationships remain in the person's mind and are continually reinforced by media, peer group and many other sources of sexuality construction long after the physical means of expression of such ideas is possible.

Sexual experience is full of hazards for us all; most of us can remember our clumsy, anxiety ridden, early sexual encounters. Sexuality after serious injury involves the same fears, uncertainties and ineptitudes as early adolescence. A person with a disability, however, is not starting ex nihilo, but must negate all previous knowledge of his or her body and social prescriptions about sexual performance in order to learn new ways of giving and receiving pleasure. To repossess the body in this intimate sense, and to share its secrets with another person is clearly a critical aspect of reconstruction of the self. Such vulnerability can of course lead to despair, but it can also constitute a significant core around which a new body image is forged. Emotional risk taking removes the person from the protective haven of patient status and propels him or her into the real world of satisfactions and sorrows—the healthy world of intimate and emotional relationships.

Spinally-injured women fare better than their male counterparts, in that they retain their fertility. They are usually still able to conceive and give birth to children. Men, however, may have difficulty obtaining an erection and ejaculation, resulting in impaired fertility (Trieschman, 1980). Lack of sensation and motor function alters the amount of pleasure experienced by both men and women, but in terms of the functional possibilities of sexual performance women fare better than men (Stewart, 1981:348). A major role of the family is to produce children, a function that is underpinned by strong cultural expectations about reproduction.

Couples who find that they are incapable of having children may feel unfulfilled.

Spinally-injured men have two types of erections—reflex and psychogenic. Reflex erections are associated with upper motor neuron, spastic injuries and occur in up to 90 percent of men with such lesions; ejaculation, however, is rare. Psychogenic erections occur with lower motor neuron, flaccid lesions; about 30 percent of males with this impairment have erections. Unlike reflex erections, which require local contact, psychogenic erections are the response to cortical activity involving vision and fantasy. Some of these men may have emissions of sperm (Stewart, 1981:348).

The possibilities of penile erection at will and ejaculation of viable sperm cells is thus very unlikely for the paralysed man. His participation in penile–vaginal intercourse and in the conception of a child has radically changed. Certainly technical developments in prosthetics and electrostimulation may bring hope to some people (Stewart, 1981:348), and modern reproductive technologies may present new opportunities for previously impotent men. The central meaning of sexuality and reproduction for the person himself, however, has been critically altered. Such practical strategies may have important functional significance, but can never ameliorate the impact of these critical bodily losses for the person concerned.

Among spinally-injured women, menstruation usually resumes two to three months after the initial trauma (Stewart, 1981:347). A paralysed woman can participate in vaginal intercourse, and although her experience of this sexual encounter has radically changed, she can conceive a child in this manner, and she can produce a healthy baby from her own damaged body. Both the potentiality and the actuality of child bearing are clearly of considerable significance. A woman can fulfill the most important tenet of femininity—she can become a mother. Moreover, the production of a child is an overt sign to others of her continuing sexuality. She must engage in a sexual act to conceive a child, her female hormones and secretions have supported this conception, her uterus has carried the developing foetus, and her damaged body has given birth to a new, healthy, living body from its disordered interior. Birth of any kind always has an element of the miraculous. The advent of new life arising out of the ruins of a damaged body contains all the elements of phoenix–like transcendence.

In many ways, then, women have a definite advantage over men in that they can produce children. Although they also experience severe alterations in sensation, paraplegic women may be seen as less disadvantaged than similarly disabled men because their sexual performance does not depend on an erect penis, and the sensations of their breasts are likely to be retained, depending on the level of the lesion.

But motherhood involves more than just giving birth to a baby. Pregnancy and lactation are clearly biologically determined. Motherhood, on the other hand, is a complex social construction that includes many gender–specific elements. Many people assume that because women give birth and lactate that women should also be the principal nurturers of children—that child bearing and child rearing are part of the same biologically determined process. It is this aspect of motherhood—the social construction of motherhood in contrast to the biological reality of pregnancy and childbirth—that can still be seriously detrimental to a paralysed woman. It is not enough just to give birth, no matter how miraculous that must be for a woman with a disordered body. In order to fulfill the primary tenet of femininity, the woman must also rear that child.

Motherhood involves a huge range of physically demanding tasks associated with cleaning, toileting, lifting, bathing, washing, playing and food preparation, which may be impossible for a woman with a disabled body. The sexual division of labour—the definition of tasks as women's work and men's work—is neither universal nor consistent, yet it can seriously discriminate against the woman with a disability and mitigate against her sense of fulfillment as a woman in a particular social context. Yet, paradoxically, this same social construction may also restrict a woman's possibilities for participation in the workforce since a woman's 'natural' role is seen as a dependent wife and mother. The rhetoric that a woman's rightful place is in the home, that her natural work is housework and childcare is clearly articulated in times of high unemployment, but at other times it is only barely hidden from view. If such ideological attitudes restrict work opportunities for ablebodied women, the effect of such strong social injunctions on the potential for disabled women to re-enter the workforce is formidable.

While the reconstitutive benefits of sexual and reproductive activities for a person with a disability may be immense, many difficulties exist beyond the physical impediments to sexual practices already discussed. Active sexual participation involves

What is health after disease or trauma? 113

finding a compatible partner, an activity fraught with emotional hazards, or renegotiating new parameters for a previously-established relationship, which may be no less difficult.

Women have a long history as carers of others. Whether married or single, women are chiefly responsible for the physical and emotional tasks of looking after other people. In formal and informal situations, in paid and unpaid labour, it is women who look after children, elderly relatives, the sick and those people who cannot take care of themselves. It is this aspect of women's role, their responsiveness to the physical and emotional needs of others, that extorts such high costs from women in terms of their own physical and emotional wellbeing and in terms of lost alternative possibilities. Middle-class women who can afford to pay other women to help with cleaning, ironing and childcare tasks fare better than working-class women who have less resources to modify the burden of their caring role, yet few women escape the formidable obligations of domestic responsibility and the care and nurturance of others.

What then is the impact of this aspect of women's gender role on men and womens' search for a partner with whom to share sexual, procreative or residential relationships? Although a paralysed woman is likely to be much less physically disabled in terms of sexuality and reproductive activities than a man with a similar injury, she may find that her ability to attract a heterosexual partner has greatly diminished because of this aspect of gender socialisation. Women are carers, men are cared for. The woman with a disability appears to need care, she does not look as though she can give care to others. A paralysed person will always be dependent on others, although for many people such dependence may be extremely minor. Others must attend to and be responsive to his or her needs. Clearly such need is inconsistent with femininity and contradictory to the ideology of women's central role as carers of others. Paralysed men are thus much more likely to develop relationships with able-bodied women; a paralysed woman is unlikely to find a long lasting partnership with an able-bodied man. The sexual and reproductive potential of paralysed women is thus subsumed by the ideology of women's role as practical carers and emotional nurturers of others, particularly men. This conflation must be a bitter irony for women with damaged bodies, and constitute a serious impediment to the full transformation of the paralysed patient to a healthy woman again.

Gender, however, is far more than just the physical aspects of sexual practice and reproduction. A man who becomes a paraplegic may find that his body will no longer enable him to do the work that he did previously. In our society work is an important aspect of life, and a critical avenue for the development of self-esteem and identity. His relationship with this major source of income and identity-production has been challenged. The paralysed man will find that his ability to sustain his masculinity through the central tenets of maleness—work, sexuality and fatherhood—can no longer be assumed.

But a vital area remains by which the paraplegic man may reconstitute his masculinity. Through energetic attention to body-building, basketball, archery and many other physical activities that involve the strong muscular work of the upper trunk, shoulder and arm muscles, the paralysed man may create a powerful physical definition of masculinity, which may override the other domains in which his masculinity is threatened. The energy and competence involved in creating the image of a paraplegic athlete, and the competitiveness and skill of wheelchair sports are powerful facilitative means for those paraplegic men who choose that path to rehabilitation—a choice unfortunately not open to quadriplegic men.

What, then, of paralysed women? Paraplegic women, like paraplegic men, gain important functional advantages from exercise, body-building and wheelchair athletics. But such activities do not have the same powerful effect for women as they do for men since such bodily attributes are associated with masculinity and are considered to be contradictory aspects of femininity. To be a women is to be passive, responsive, attractive and a mother (Oakley, 1981). Bodily exercise is undertaken by women for important functional reasons—to keep fit, to prevent pressure sores, to transfer from chair to bed and to other locations. More critically, women exercise in order to hold off the visual effects of paralysed muscles for as long as possible, to keep slim, and to retain a good posture. Yet such efforts may be a losing battle in the face of the inevitability of muscle loss. Women may be seen as doubly handicapped: first by their actual physical loss, and secondly by the high value society places on female appearance and body shape (Campling, 1979).

Thus gender—the social construction of masculinity and femininity—weaves a confusing web for disabled men and women. Unexpected traps await the body, contradictory messages confuse the mind. Yet these profound alterations in bodily performance, appearance and sensation provide valuable insights

What is health after disease or trauma?   115

into taken for granted aspects of gender-role socialisation in general, and the influence of such ideology on our own relationships with others. A paralysed woman loses less in terms of sexual performance and her potential to bear a child. Such possibilities may amount to pyrrhic victories, however, since dominant tenets of womanhood in our society may deny her the opportunity to enjoy this potential. While her non-normal appearance may not deter more pragmatic contact, the appearance of a wheelchair is an unequivocal sign of permanent disability and is likely to preclude the possibilities of intimate relationship. Even the woman's ability to conceive and give birth to a child—to be a mother—is held in uneasy tension with the assumption of her diminished ability to nurture and care for others—the essence of motherhood.

While the paralysed man has far less physical potential for sexual fulfillment and fatherhood, he has at least two significant avenues for the reconstitution of self open to him, which provide him with considerable advantages over a similarly disabled woman. Through exercise and sport, the paraplegic man can construct a bodily presentation of masculinity, which has currency in the able-bodied world—it is an exterior image that is valued in the real world and has the potential to override the aspects of masculinity he has lost. Secondly, men are traditionally the objects of womens' care and nurture. This important aspect of gender, which is detrimental to a disabled woman's rehabilitation as a mother and as a sexual partner, presents much more positive opportunities to a man. A man is much more likely to be cared for by a woman in an institutional setting and such experience will enhance his opportunities for finding a woman to care for him in his reconstituted life in the everyday world. Gender in this context, as in the wider society, is not an equal opportunity phenomenon.

How does the paralysed person select a satisfactory new conception of self? Relevance is a crucial issue for the problems I address here. Not everything present in a situation is relevant to the patient. How does the patient choose from the myriad of ideas that flood into his or her world?

Some factors in a situation impose themselves upon the actor. Schutz calls these factors imposed relevances (Wagner, 1970: 113). Other issues are selected out by the individual as important to him or her now. These Schutz calls volitional or intrinsic relevances (Wagner, 1970:113). Severe body paralysis is imposed on the individual. The individual must concern him or herself to understand the problem. But to do this he or she must define what the problem is. The enormity of the physical loss is of central relevance for the patient. The loss becomes the theme of his or her cognitive efforts, but the physical loss will be differentially perceived by different people, depending on their various previous interests.

Severe body paralysis is a new and unknown experience for the patient. The person's previous interests seem to have little relevance to this new body state. The situation is filled with uncertainty. The past, it seems, has little relevance for the present or the future. A new interpretation is needed to fit the problem into the larger context of the patient's knowledge that relates to the problem. The elements a person may select from his or her stock of knowledge as important for this task are called by Schutz interpretational relevances. The patient sorts out his or her given knowledge in relation to the new problem, the physical loss.

The voluntary nature of this selection, however, must not be overestimated. Not only has the patient's physical loss imposed a set of relevances upon the person, but the institutional venue for the rehabilitation has circumscribed further boundaries of relevance. The paralysed person is still a member of the social world. The established social systems of relevance of the wider community further constrain the selection of a satisfactory new conception of self. The paralysed person must orient him or herself to the existing values of the cultural group. The individual is free to choose, but only within the limits prescribed by these imposed relevances. The way each person recognises what is socially relevant is through an understanding of the social system of typifications and relevances—through knowledge of his or her culture.

So, for the task of reconstruction, the patient selects materials from two main sources: from past experiences and knowledge, and from an understanding of his or her social context. Personal thematic and interpretational relevances are oriented to past understandings of the self and to present understandings of the social world.

Another issue that must be considered in the context of the reconstitution of health is motivation. In everyday usage, the word motivation is used to refer to several quite different processes. Schutz insisted that the subjective meaning of motives must be distinguished from their objective meaning. Schutz distinguished between 'in-order-to' motives and 'because' motives (Schutz, 1972:86ff). An in-order-to motive refers to the actor's intention to bring about a projected goal during the process of its ongoing action. As such, an in-order-to motive has a subjective meaning; it cannot be perceived by the outside observer. When the action has been completed, however, the actor may turn back to these past actions as an observer of him or herself and explore the reasons why those choices were made. The genuine because motive is an objective category, accessible to the outside observer. The because motive is the reason people give for their actions. It is anchored in the past: it relates to past lived experiences. The meaning context of the true because motive is always an explanation after the event.

Once completed, action appears as though it were a unity from original project to completion. The multiplicity and complexity of its component phases are lost from the vantage point of the backward glance. The actor may claim that he or she selected this course of action in preference to that course of action in order to bring about a chosen goal. But this claim is an interpretation of the past. An interpretation of the past is determined by the 'Here and Now' in which the actor now stands. The choice of which past experiences are to be regarded as the genuine because motive of the original project depends on the cone of light ego lets fall on its experience preceding the project (Schutz, 1972:95). Because motives are '...simply memories that have received their perspective, their horizons, their highlights and shadows, from a Here and Now always later than the one in which the project was constituted' (Schutz, 1972:95).

I have taken some time to explore the dangers inherent in any attempt to reconstruct a biography. In order to look back on what has gone before one must deal in because motives. This is right and proper. Because motives are anchored in the past: they relate to past lived experiences. But the past is interpreted by the actor in terms of his or her present interest. Acting in the present, the actor attributes a preliminary understanding to a certain event in the past. The person sees his or her action as a choice between several possible actions, and once chosen, the action is seen as a performed unity between conception and completion. Interpretation of past events depends on where the actor now stands. But where the actor now stands depends on a sedimentation of knowledge, experience and meaning over many years. The issues an actor selects as relevant are determined by his or her interests prevailing at a particular time. To focus on

118   Bodily alterations

because motives as explanation, without an awareness of the emergent and processual composition of their reality, is to seriously distort the relationship between the past and the present in the actor's social world.

The reconstruction of biography is an endeavour fraught with difficulties for the sociological investigator too. The documentary method is used by the investigator to construct a life history for another. Past occurrences are selected and ordered by the investigator to furnish the patient's condition, its relevant past and future prospects (Garfinkel, 1962:705). Not only must the investigator 'manage situations' in various ways outlined by Garfinkel, but always within an additional set of conditions relating to the knowledge that his or her actions and products will be subject to review by others and must be justified to them. Discussion of sociological methods rarely recognises the fact that sociological inquiries are 'carried out under common sense auspices at the points where decisions about the correspondence between observed appearances and intended events are being made' (Garfinkel, 1962:709). While the advocates of scientific research denounce the subjective bias of the documentary method of information gathering, they ignore the objective illusion embodied in their own methodology (Lally and Preston, 1973).

The retrospective reading of social action thus presents problems at two levels: at the level of the social actor, and at the level of the investigator of the social actor. With this in mind, I present the following data. Previous conceptions of health, given to me in retrospect by my informants, are juxtaposed against their present conceptions of health. Some of my respondents were injured twenty years previously, other less than three months. Corroboration by different informants at different stages of recovery and rehabilitation has helped my understanding of the information given to me. The preceding lengthy discussion was a necessary prerequisite for understanding the constitution of the data I now present.

Competitive sport was not only Jim's full-time career and leisure-time activity, sport was Jim's life before his paralysis. 'I was infatuated with sport. Sport was my identity. It made me a person.' Health the fitness were aspects of his conception of self that he took for granted. 'People who were not involved in sport were nobody. They didn't really exist. They were just hanging around. I couldn't understand what they were doing anyway.'

Jim played paraplegic sport for a time, but didn't really enjoy it. 'I never identified with them.' Yet Jim's previous preoccupation with sport was the element around which his transformed conception of health was moulded. Jim has reinserted himself into his old sporting world—a world devoted to young, fit and physically-oriented people, seemingly the antithesis of his present physical condition. His involvement with the management side of the sport he once played has been a satisfactory medium through which to reconstitute his conception of self. Enough of his former environment persists to present a sense of continuity. His incapacity for involvement at one level of the sport has been substituted for an energetic involvement at another level. Health exists for Jim in his busy life. But health has been transformed for him by his passage through a disease context.

Phillip, like Jim, was strongly oriented toward competitive sport and an outdoor life. He had achieved high status in various competitive sports, and did not consider that he had reached the height of his sporting career. To be fit and healthy—to be able to engage in competitive sport—was for Phillip 'a way of life; a state of mind.' Phillip claims that 'being paralysed would be a big drag if you were not able to work, and were not interested in sport.' Phillip has had to reorient his interests, but he has not had to reduce his activities. At the time of writing, Phillip has been a paraplegic for only a year. Although he will not be able to continue the apprenticeship programme in which he was engaged, he has already found a place in a business owned by a relation. Paraplegic sports will not seem second best to his previous involvement in national level sport, but rather will present 'another challenge'. Phillip says, 'I have become the person I was before the accident'. For an enthusiastic, topflight sportsman like Phillip, the meaning of health has been transformed. Yet health exists, with enough elements from a previous conception to present a sense of continuity.

Pam, too, was a highly competitive sportswoman before her accident. She was always very conscious of her figure, and took plenty of exercise. Being healthy for Pam was having the energy to play the sport, engage in many extra activities, as well as looking after her house and three young children. Pam conceives of herself now as very healthy. 'I lead a very stimulating life. My family have never accepted that there is anything I can't do. The only thing they will accept is that I can't go up steps.' She considered that it took at least three years before she was 'confident of myself and my ability to understand what I was—this is a matter of experience.' Pam says she is much more conscious of her body now. She watches what she eats and drinks, and is constantly alert to areas of her body she can't feel.

Although Michael was not involved in competitive sport in the same sense as Jim, Phillip and Pam, he had strong and definite ideas about his own health. Michael was very involved in body building. He had definite ideas about the body shape he considered right for himself. Proper shape included 'a decent set of arms, good shoulders and chest. I never was much of a one for developed leg muscles'. He saw his body-building exercises as important for both his occupation as a construction worker and his leisure interests. But the aesthetic aspect of a strong, well-developed shoulder, girdle and chest was of great importance to Michael's conception of himself.

Michael's previous emphasis on the top half of his body has been a lucky coincidence for his new body state. 'All my life, everything has been arms, chest, shoulders, stomach. Legs were just there to carry me around. Legs got me in the right position to enable me to do the rest. Legs were just the technical part. These parts of my body (indicating chest and arms) were what I needed most. Now I need them even more.' Physical appearance was an important element in Michael's previous conception of self. Happily his previous de-emphasis of the lower extremities in favour of the upper extremities has stood him in good stead for becoming a paraplegic. Although it is early days yet, Michael's projection of himself into the future includes a paying job, an independent living situation and a goal of championship paraplegic sport.

Frank was used to hard physical labour both on his farm and also when he went shearing for other farmers. Although he took his health for granted, he considered himself extremely fit. Frank feels frustrated at the limited number of activities he can do as a high-level quadriplegic. He finds it difficult to dissipate his energy. He has rejected a motorised chair, because pushing a wheelchair helps a little to this end. He regrets that he has no interest in some of the usual activities for quadriplegic people, such as painting with the brush held between the teeth. 'Some people get a lot of pleasure doing these things. But they were probably oriented to doing these things before. I consider myself fit now, but I no longer take my health for granted. Before I could give myself a thrashing and get over it. Now I am very cautious and careful with my body. I know now what the problem is. I know what has to be done. I consider myself absolutely

What is health after disease or trauma?

a person. I am handicapped, but I have a mind of my own. I am able to choose what I want.'

Although Bob had never played competitive sport, he saw himself as a 'fitness freak'. His occupation as a seaman demanded a high degree of physical fitness. Bob exercised and ran regularly. Although his health had never been challenged, Bob was always concerned to maintain the degree of fitness that satisfied his conception of himself.

Both Jim and Bob are severely paralysed. But the job opportunities allocated to them by vocational guidance officers were quite at variance with the way they saw themselves. Bob was given a typewriter by the vocational worker and told to move the carriage. He said, 'But I don't want to typewrite. Give me the money. I want to run a business'. Bob never heard from the agency again. He did, in fact, develop a small business, entirely without professional help. Jim was taken daily, in a marked bus, to a sheltered workshop where he was put to work in the bootmaker's shop. 'Cobbling was probably a noble art, a respected way of life. But I don't want to be a cobbler.' Jim, too, has subsequently developed a very satisfactory occupational career for himself, a career vastly different from that proposed by the vocational officer.

'Living is the most important thing: treatment and medical care follow this.' Although Bob's initial hospitalisation was at least two years, this maxim has influenced the way he sees himself ever since. Bob is virtually a total quadriplegic. His paralysis is the result of poliomyelitis, so is slightly patchy, yet he pursues a workday life that would make many able-bodied people wilt. In addition he is involved in many committees and a full family life, including three children.

Unlike the other people I have mentioned, Maggie had no particular area of physical expertise. She loved walking, watched her diet and considered herself 'normally healthy'. Maggie also says she is much more aware of her own body now. Now she reacts to symptoms that previously she would have ignored.

Conceptual reorientation is not determined by the physical changes people experience, nor from pre-existing personality characteristics. New meanings emerge from the ongoing processes. Each new event poses new problems, which require new interpretations and new definitions of the situation. Re-evaluations of past relevances and future anticipations are woven into the ongoing stream of meaning and experience.

By its very presence a disordered body challenges the status quo, and in so doing it may illuminate possibilities, point to new realities, and suggest that the routines of everyday life may not be immutable. Despite the many physical, conceptual, emotional and social barriers that have been explored, many people with severe bodily alterations do come to see themselves as healthy. The transformation of a patient to a healthy person again is a triumphant victory.

Yet a death has occurred; and it is critical that this death is acknowledged. The body has undergone major alterations. It is not the same body. The body has been estranged from the self. The person has experienced disembodiment. The person's new transformed concept of health has arisen from the ruins of his or her old self. Although significant strands from the past have been drawn into the new conception, many elements of the new healthy self have derived from the ongoing rehabilitation processes. Knowledge, meanings and understandings about the old body have passed away. A new self has risen from the ashes of the old body.

Continuity of self-conception was so often claimed as to be almost an act of faith amongst many of my informants. The reasons for such claims are not hard to understand. To profess that nothing has changed may provide a sense of social stability during a phase of enormous change. But to insist that the person has not changed, that he or she is the same person, is to bind the person into a dysfunctional illusion—an illusion that will continuously present the person with irrelevant and unfulfillable goals. By imprisoning the mind in the possibilities of the past, such claims may inhibit the discovery of new meanings and possibilities for the future. These claims deny the fact that the meaning of health for the person has been transformed. Failure to acknowledge such a serious disruption trivialises the disembodiment and reduces the enormity of the rehabilitation tasks for the person with serious bodily alterations. But such assertions are also socially reassuring. People can continue to relate to the person as though nothing has happened. Such strategies prevent awkwardness, they allow polite social interaction to continue. Others do not have to contemplate the inconceivable reality of permanent bodily loss. Such interaction does not challenge the status quo, no threatening possibilities can arise. But to treat the person as though nothing has happened denies the person the reality of his or her body, and may ultimately be just as destructive to the person as directly focussing on the bodily changes.

Exploration of the disruption of identity experienced by a person with serious bodily alterations provides insights into many other personal and social transformations. Certainly visible body changes are the most dangerous catalysts of self-deconstruction. Disease or injury involving loss of a part of the body such as an amputation, or changes in external appearance such as scarring, hair loss or severe skin rashes may present difficulties for many people, but additions to the body such as prostheses, colostomy bags, joint replacements, mammary and facial reconstructions can also provoke grief for the loss of a person's former self-concept. Other more general physiological alterations such as dementia, ageing and menopause may also fit the analysis presented here. Dementia is a particularly interesting contrast to the severe bodily losses that have been the focus of this study. Dementia is often referred to as a living death; what has died is not the body but the ability of the mind to form a conceptualisation of the self. Dementia is an expression of a profound irony: the body is complete, healthy and intact, the mind has become detached from the living body.

Menopause is another bodily change that can evoke tension and anxiety. Menopause brings a woman's reproductive life to an end. If being a mother is central to femininity, the physiological fact that a woman can no longer be a mother is an issue of social significance, and thus of personal concern. the body has changed, it is no longer capable of reproduction. With such powerful social constructions of feminity it is not surprising that many women feel that they are no longer 'real women' after menopause occurs—that this physiological event heralds the end of relevant life and the beginning of the asexuality of old age. Even those women who rejoice that the cycle of menstruation is over grieve for this reassuring sign of their reproductive potential—their womanliness.

The 'mid-life crisis' in men, erroneously called the male menopause, has been raised to the status of a syndrome in recent years. Although the term is somewhat amorphous, the central issues in this male crisis are related to the person's perceptions of changes in the appearance and capacities of his body, grief for unconsummated potential, and anticipatory sorrow for the diminished ability of the body to cope with the future. If the man should experience a heart attack at this time, such a clinical event further reinforces the man's loss of faith in his body. The body is fallible; it has let him down. The potential for fulfillment previously displayed by the outward bodily signs of masculinity such as force, competence and assertiveness gives way to the appearance of old age and the implications of sexual, political and social impotence that such signs signify in our society.

Our body is the core of all understanding about ourselves and our place in the world. We are obsessed with our bodies. We have no other means of knowing ourselves. We experience the world through our bodies. We use our bodies as a resource in order to derive meaning from experiences and events. Through using our body as a resource we construct, over time, a sense of our body as being—our self-body identity. We, quite literally, cannot think ourselves beyond our bodies. We cannot ignore or hold off, we cannot bypass or avoid our bodies because we need our bodies in order to develop our ideas about the world and our place in society. We use our bodies to discover the world, the social world in turn imposes its classifications and categories, its customs and approved behaviours on our body. The liaison is absolute, Separation is unthinkable. The relationship between the body and society is the structure of our self, the substance of our awareness and our view of the world.

This corporeal preoccupation makes us extremely vulnerable to degradations, deteriorations and alterations of the body. Bodily changes and alterations are dangerous. They threaten the bond between the self, the body and society. Severe body alterations of the kind which have been the focus of this study represent a threat to the established order. The person is likely to be male, young, at least initially, and of intact intelligence. His or her body has been severed from its social and personal moorings. The body has, in a sense, asserted its supremacy over society. The body has rebelled against the disciplines and routines of childhood learning. Unless checked, the person could devise new strategies for his or her body which might not conform to socially approved modes of bodily behaviour and action. Rehabilitation, resocialisation in a rehabilitation unit, can be seen as the endeavor to resocialise the dangerous elements of the anarchic body—to recivilise the body—which has escaped from its social bonds.

Rehabilitation is the reimposition of society on the body; the relearning of socially appropriate behaviour for paraplegic and quadriplegic people, for ageing people, for people who have had heart attacks, for people with inflammatory arthritis. The rehabilitation unit is a specialist domain removed from the everyday world, the real world of values and hierarchies, of politics and relationships. Resocialisation in this domain may have little currency in terms of the values of the everyday world. The transformative triumphs of a paralysed person who sees him or herself as healthy again must be balanced against the personal and social losses that have accrued in the passage through a patient status. Activities, appearances and opportunities that may be raised as evidence of good recovery and excellent rehabilitation may have little or no value in terms of the everyday world. Disabled people who do succeed in meeting the goals of the wider society may be seen to be not truly representative of a particular disability, but to be an exception. An uneasy tension exists between holding on to the past, with its association with positive values, or renegotiating a new, more appropriate reality, with its potential for negative connotations. These issues will be explored in more depth in the last chapter.

Is there health after disease? What is health for the severely paralysed person? These people see themselves as healthy. Their ideas of health have undergone radical change. Their reconstituted healthy selves accommodate elements quite different from those of their formerly healthy selves. A sense of continuity is preserved by the emergent nature of the transformational process. By redefinitions, re-evaluations and retrospective reconstructions, the past is made to fit the future. Ideas and bodily states that would previously have been inconsistent with a person's self-conception of health are now incorporated into a new, ongoing, but transformed conception of health.

The maintenance of this new conception can never be taken for granted. It is a fragile social construction, susceptible to new relevances that can alter the balance of its constitutive elements. But for now, and for the individual, health exists and invests his or her experience with meaning.

10 Rehabilitation— the dilemmas

Social order and stability are attained by the gradual process of taming the body, of constraining the natural desires of the body to conform to social patterns of behaviour. Through training and learning the human body is transformed into a social body. We learn to know about our bodies, and what to do with our bodies in order to be good citizens. Society provides us with the structures and the categories, the language and the behaviours which enable us to make sense of our bodies and to use our bodies in a socially approved manner. Our body is the resource by which we learn about other aspects of society. Our eyes perceive, our ears hear, our organs conform and our limbs reach out to explore and discover the environments in which we live. The human body is thoroughly embedded within the social body; it is only through society that we may understand and give meaning to the experiences of our body.

As we grow up we learn from others how our body should behave in particular situations. Such learning is difficult at first, but eventually the body is subdued and the activity, be it hunger, micturition, defaecation or sleep becomes routinised; we no longer think about it or if we do we assume that such regulation is natural—that having three meals a day, sleeping for eight hours at night, urinating only in a defined place are natural, not social, imperatives. The body is captured by society. A person demonstrates maturity by the manner in which he or she deploys his or her body to others, in both private and public domains.

Alterations to the body in later life challenge this lifetime process of bodily constraint. In a sense, the body re-asserts its supremacy over society—it escapes from its social bonds. Carefully established patterns of body regulation and conformity are threatened; the body rebels against its social regulation: past learning is rendered problematic. But such alterations in function, movement and appearance also threaten social order. Disordered activities in a mature body threaten our tenuous complacency in our bodies and in society. The body has escaped its social shackles; years of careful socialisation are rendered null and void. Civilised life is threatened by the very existence of a disordered body. The anarchic presence of the body mocks the civilising forces of social constraint.

Rehabilitation reconstitutes social order. Through the processes of rehabilitation the anarchic body is brought to heel, the body is recivilised. The potential chaos of the uncivilised body is subordinated by a wide variety of institutional imperatives. The body is resocialised—it is reordered to conform to the imperatives of the wider society.

But the imperatives of the wider society may no longer be appropriate to the person's new body capabilities. The rehabilitation team may work hard to resocialise the person's damaged body to fit a society to which the person can never aspire.

Rehabilitation is no simple assembly line process of body restoration. The human body, unlike a mechanical body, defies such didactic prescriptions. The human body is not an entity unto itself. The body itself cannot be worked on in isolation. The body is bound in partnership with the mind, and each is embedded within the wider society in which the person lives. The triumvirate is fundamental. The body cannot be perceived except by means of the mind, the mind cannot designate meaning except through the categories provided by society. This is the bond that is shattered by disease and trauma.

As soon as body changes can be seen in terms of this bond, the dilemmas inherent in rehabilitation, as a practice within the paradigm of medicine, become apparent. Physical rehabilitation is critical work, but it is only a part of a much larger project— the reconstitution of the individual's identity within the wider social world. Narrow definitions of rehabilitation restrict the possibilities of change; by ignoring the cognitive and social dimensions of the body such definitions seriously detract from the restoration of self after bodily alterations. By failing to acknowledge the central importance of these dimensions of genuine rehabilitation, people with disordered bodies are consigned to the impossible task of self-restoration without accounting for the handicapping and facilitative effects of the past, of significant others and of society's structural impediments. We set people up to fail, and we blame them when, inevitably, they do.

The spinal unit is a medical domain especially instituted to manage bodily losses, disabilities and malfunctions. The institution works on the parts of the body in order to develop alternative movements and methods of control. The destruction, however, is permanent.

At a time selected by the institution the body is declared rehabilitated. The person may now graduate into the everyday world, with the directive to act normally like everyone else. Having worked extensively on the body of the paralysed person, the institution now asks that the person disattends to his or her body. The person is asked to transcend his or her body in order to re-enter society on the same terms as everyone else.

Not only does the institution direct the paralysed person to assimilate, to disregard his or her bodily losses, but it expects that the public will also disregard the visible signs of abnormality. Cultural definitions of normalcy are strongly influenced by medicine. Yet medicine asks the public to suspend these definitions when it suits them in order to further a rehabilitative project begun in a medical domain. Family and formerly significant others are asked to accept as unchanged someone who has in fact become radically changed.

In severe body paralysis the actual physical loss is the primary agent of transformation of identity. But institutional imperatives and organisational logic play a large part in the deconstitution of self which occurs in the passage of a person to a patient. The spinal unit is a paraplegic world. Yet the goal of the rehabilitation procedures in this world is to inject the paralysed person back into the non-paraplegic, everyday world. Having instituted procedures to transform the person into a patient, to establish his or her non-normalcy, the institution then pushes the paralysed person out into the world insisting that he or she is normal like everyone else.

It is undeniable that the reassimilation of paralysed people into the everyday world of work, play, family and social relationships is a desirable ideal. But the directive to assimilate, to act normally like everyone else, can be seriously discriminatory. The quadriplegic and paraplegic peron is not normal like everyone else. The body does not move like other people's bodies; the organs do not function in the same way. The self is not in the normal packaging; normal modes of expression are not available.

Another dilemma facing the paralysed person may be equally discriminatory. The influence of the spinal unit is strong, and continues throughout the paralysed person's life. The dedication and enthusiasm of the coordinated team of professional workers is not challenged. But the values, assumptions and expectations of the members of the specialist domain can present a formidable barrier to the development of a satisfactory new self-identity for the paralysed person.

Quadriplegia and paraplegia most often occur in young people, people with most of their lives before them. These people come from a wide range of social classes, ages and interest groups. The strongly articulated rehabilitative goals of sport, work, assimilation and social usefulness may be irrelevant to the individual paralysed person. In a crisis of such dimensions, the temptation to tell people how to run their lives, and to set guidelines of ideal behaviour is well intentioned and hard to resist. Sympathetic workers suggest well tried avenues of rehabilitation in an effort not to perpetuate or add to the catastrophe.

But the basis of the helping professions must be that the person is free to accept or refuse help. The person has needs, values and standards of behaviour that may not be shared, but that must be seen as legitimate. The recently paralysed person requires expert help to restore function and control. But the mandate to work on parts of the body should not be assumed to include control over a person's life. Central to rehabilitation must be the idea that the person is still free, as he or she always was, to make choices and to take the consequences for those choices. That these choices may not relate to the goals of the rehabilitation unit is inconsequential. The paralysed person has no obligation to accept things as they are because 'this is the best way now' or because 'this is the way things have always been.'

Despite their physical disabilities many paralysed people do become useful citizens, do hold important jobs, do achieve great merit in sporting and other activities. The enormous handicaps that must be overcome to achieve such successes must not be minimised. But not everyone values these achievements, nor sees these goals in relationship to his or her own identity. The undeniable physical benefit of work and active participation in sport must be separated from its central, value-laden position in emotional adjustment, coping and psychological acceptance of physical loss.

It is the task of the rehabilitation team to demonstrate the physical advantages of a regular routine, of active participation in sport, of techniques of bladder and bowel management and pressure sore prevention. But to invest these practical techniques with emotional value and social merit is wrong. Vocational rehabilitation, musculoskeletal rehabilitation, rehabilitation of the urogenital tract are essential, practical tasks. But the sum of these individual rehabilitative tasks must not be seen as the total rehabilitation of the paralysed man or woman. Rehabilitation—the confluence of identity and the new body state—can only be done by the person him or herself, in his or her own time, and in terms of the society in which he or she must live. The goal of rehabilitation in a spinal injuries unit is to teach the paralysed person to manage the loss of movement and control, but the goal of rehabilitation itself is far wider. It relates to the specific concerns of the paralysed person, and to the wider issue of the relationship of the body to interaction and identity formation in the context of the society in which the person lives.

In order to accomplish the gargantuan task of disattending to the body, the paralysed person is expected to show great courage, determination and will power. Should these efforts fail to impress others, the paralysed person is accused of having a deficient personality, of lack of motivation, or of moral inadequacy. The often repeated phrases, that an experience with quadriplegia or paraplegia can make you a 'better person', a 'worthwhile citizen', a 'useful member of society', reflect this same suggestion of responsibility on the part of the paralysed person. Why should the disabled person be expected to be useful? We have no more right to demand this of a paralysed person than we have to demand it of each other.

How do quadriplegic or paraplegic people deal with these dilemmas? Not only must they come to terms with these imposed values and expectations, but they must also re-enter a world that does not see them as normal and is not organised in terms of their needs.

Assimilation and integration are much used and much misunderstood words. They most often refer simply to accommodation within the community, as opposed to within an institution. Little thought is given to the quality of the assimilated life. This place in the community is vulnerable, since it depends on the goodwill of others. The everyday world provides some refuges for the disabled. The 'brave paraplegic', 'the cripple battling against all odds' are culturally available models of disabled identity that paralysed people may choose to accept. These cultural models are legitimated by the everyday world. They may provide great comfort and shelter to paralysed people. Yet the parameters of such cultural identities are strictly defined in terms of the normal world. Acceptance by the world on these terms may severely confine the processes of identity construction and modes of expression available to a disabled person. So long as paralysed people can disattend to their bodies and present themselves as normal, they may gain acceptance in the world. They must be grateful to be allowed to participate in the real world, to accept the goodwill of others, but they are not free to question or refuse for fear of losing hard won gains. The needs and possibilities of paralysed people remain privatised and fragmented.

Failure is embedded into the very principles of rehabilitation. By tying people to their past and by projecting goals suited to the able-bodied world, rehabilitation workers deny the reality of disembodiment—of self-body dislocation—and unwittingly mystify the rehabilitation process for those people with altered bodies.

Rehabilitation workers are, of course, members of the everyday world and are thus subject to its categories. Although they have learned specialised techniques of bodily restoration in training schools, they also operate with many commonsense understandings about disability and rehabilitation. The problem is not that rehabilitation workers are capable, as we all are, of misunderstanding and wrongful interpretation, but that their expert status invests them with infallibility. We expect them to be aware of existing knowledge, we expect that they have studied the personal and social meaning of body loss, and we expect that they will use this knowledge and understanding in the best interests of the person with a disability.

A recent survey of health science students, including physiotherapists, occupational therapists, nurses and speech pathologists, many of whom will subsequently work in rehabilitation settings, showed them to have unduly narrow and pessimistic beliefs concerning the lives and problems of handicapped people (Westbrook et al., 1988:311). The students seemed more aware of the handicaps of people with more visible stigmatised and tragic disorders, and underestimated the handicaps of people with less visible disabilities, particularly those of older people. It is not hard to see that such attitudes may contribute to unrealistically low expectations for people with disabilities, inappropiate treatment plans and goals and irrelevant advice to people and their families (Westbrook et al., 1988:311). The power of rehabilitation workers to construct and control the process of rehabilitation, and the vulnerable rehabilitatee's blind faith in the workers' assumptions and expectations, are major factors leading to the frustrations expressed by many of my informants. Sexist, racist, and age-and class-based assumptions are commonplace, but the rehabilitation worker's expert status invests these discriminatory attitudes with the patina of professional knowledge.

Rehabilitation is an intensely individualistic activity. The individual is isolated from his or her past and present interactive environment. The rehabilitation unit, the finite meaning province of the patient, seems distinct and removed from the world of everyday life. The intensive focus on body work is detached from the person's self-constitution in his or her biographical past, and remote from the concerns of the everyday world. This focus deepens and perpetuates the disembodiment caused by the initial trauma or disease. The unrelenting focus of attention on the disordered body denies the person's past and lived experience; it reduces the body to an object separate from its self-apprehension and social insertion. Such work denies the inextricable relationship between the self, the body and society; it exacerbates the alienation.

Rehabilitation is, by its very nature, a conservative endeavour. It operates within an orientation of compromise, of patching up, of making do. It encourages people to mimic the attitudes and behaviours of the world in which they can no longer compete on equal terms. It teaches people to diminish their differentness and aspire to irrelevant goals in order to appear normal. Doubtless, in the short term, this is a comforting approach. In the long term, and more generally, it must be seen as a seriously discriminatory activity. By encouraging people to compete for scarce resources on the inequitable terms of others, rehabilitation workers may commit such people to life of frustrated goals and irrelevant aspirations.

The exigent and difficult reality of quadriplegia and paraglegia encourages a tendency towards pragmatism. In the face of such devastating loss, the impulse to tell people that nothing has changed is easy to understand. But although this illusion may provide a semblance of control, workers may in fact exacerbate the alienation and increase the powerlessness of people with severe disabilities. By continuing to defer to the dictates of the status quo, people with bodily changes are persuaded to aspire to unrealistic goals, and thus to be continually frustrated by their inability to achieve them.

A more realistic approach to rehabilitation requires a brave stand on the part of the rehabilitation worker as well as the person with a disabled body. Acknowledgement of the disruption between the self and the body, and awareness of the social construction of both self-image and body experience, is an essential first step. Current rehabilitation programmes are not simple. This study has provided evidence of the complexity of such work. Yet rehabilitation in relation to the triumvirate explored in this study is vast and extends far beyond the parameters of rehabilitation as it is currently constituted. The limitations of the current model made evident by this exploration of the mind-body-society relationship point to new directions for rehabilitation, to a less manageable programme but to a more genuine attack on the enormous issue of body change as a personal loss in a social domain. The enormity of this enterprise is daunting. While clinical rehabilitation is critical and cannot be neglected, enthusiasm for rehabilitation of the body must not blind people to the broader meaning of rehabilitation—reconstitution of the self.

We have explored dominant social understandings relating to appearance, sexuality, work, masculinity, femininity and the upright posture. Such social categories may disable everyone. Yet we do not have to succumb to every aspect of such categories. We can by our actions hold off or defy some social associations. If women did not reach for the bottle of dye at the first sign of a grey hair, the negative associations with grey hair could be challenged. We collude in our own social oppression by the haste with which we attempt to disguise our bodies to conform to the stereotype of youth. Such defiance requires more than individual action of course, but the assertive power of grey hair associated with active social participation may reverse the dominant stereotype of grey hair as a symbol of asexuality, marginality and social irrelevancy, particularly in women.

Although the task is enormous, many aspects of visible disability, so long enmeshed in tragedy, bravery and invalid status can also be turned around. Professional workers can support disabled people to defy such categories. Instead of encouraging the narrowly defined, passive, apologetic lifestyles in which many people with disabilities find themselves, rehabilitation workers may empower people to break the bounds of their narrowly defined role. Just as over-protective parents shackle their children to the parameters of childhood, over-zealous rehabilitation workers may bind their clients to the confines of invalid status, the narrow half-life of disability, and preclude them from the successes and failures, the joys and sadnesses of life in the everyday world.

Rehabilitation workers overprotect disabled people by suggesting that the person is normal like everyone else. This is clearly untrue—the world does not see such people as normal. This mystification serves to bind such people to invalid status since they must aspire to unrealistic goals and will always fail to achieve success on the inequitable terms of the able-bodied world. It is only when rehabilitation workers can understand disability as a social problem, not an individual problem, and when they can approach rehabilitation from a broader social perspective (which does not exclude either the physical or the psychological) that such workers can truly help the client in the enormous task of reconstitution of self. Rather than perpetuating the illusion that people with severe disabilities are 'normal' like everyone else, rehabilitation workers can empower such people by encouraging and supporting them to defy such restrictive categories—to break the boundaries of the usual narrowly-defined roles society provides for people with these conditions.

Living is a process of change and continuous loss. By merely existing our bones and cartilages, our hair and nails, our muscles and skin grow and develop, mature and degenerate. With inexorable certitude we lose childhood when we become adolescent, we lose being nineteen when we turn twenty, we lose youth with grey hair, we lose vitality to the tuneless accompaniment of creaking joints. Biology plods a unilinear path; the effect of such biological inevitabilities is exacerbated by the social categories in which these changes are placed. All biological processes are embedded in social meaning. Knowing this releases us from the bounds of biological determinism, it points to liberty and freedom. We are no longer held captive by our genes, by our tyrannical anatomy and despotic physiological processes. What men and women have created, men and women can change.

No one claims that the task is easy. Social structures do not melt away because we fix them with our glare. The world will not automatically cleave to accommodate new categories. But acknowledgement that the established order is not immutable points to the possibilities of change—of optimism and hope in place of resignation and despair. Men and women are not trapped in the inevitabilities of biology or the changes that may be visited upon them by the vagaries of disease and injury. Men and women are bodies, but they are not just bodies; they are social beings and they have minds. These resources can bind, but they may also reveal enormous potential for change and endless new meaning. Individual experiences must be set within the broader social context in order to see that personal troubles are not unique to a particular person, but reflect the categories of the wider society.

Permanent and extensive body paralysis presents a rare opportunity to examine the relationship between the body, self identity, and society. The body, in effect, becomes separated from the identity of the paralysed person. Observation of the sociological processes which act to consolidate this separation, and subsequently to reconstitute the relationship between body and self in quadriplegic and paraplegic people, provides critical insights into these usually taken for granted processes in all social relationships. Very few, if any, of the experiences explored in this study are peculiar to people with severe disabilities. The experiences of people with quadriplegia and paraplegia exemplify in a highly visible way the same social impediments and constraints which face us all. The body is integral to all social relationships, to all understanding of ourselves and our place in the world. Certainly the primary concern for the paralysed person is that his or her body will limit his or her social possibilities. But the social world which pre-exists each individual imposes limits on what is biologically possible.

The analytically simple progression I have mapped out may make the transformative processes seem inevitable. I have attempted to present a sequential picture of change over a period of time. The end point of my analysis, a paralysed person who sees himself or herself as healthy, is an ideal that although some obtain, many do not. My study is analytical not statistical, suggestive not prescriptive. Any suggestion of simplicity of process or inevitability of the goal is due to my methodology, and does not reflect the immense physical and conceptual obstacles which these people must overcome.

The body is undoubtedly biological. Embodiment is the process whereby anatomy becomes human. Meaning is grafted onto biology by social processes. The meaning of alterations to the appearance and functioning of the body can only be understood within this same framework of contextually specific social meanings.

Exploration of established realities by sociological methods promises exciting discoveries. By challenging the inevitability of such categories and exposing their social construction, new possibilities and directions for change will become visible. The enormous personal task of rehabilitation after severe body loss will be made less difficult by illuminating the social forces that define and maintain the person as disabled, and that further handicap the already disabled person.

My effort to disestablish the taken for granted nature of social reality, at the level of personal experience and meaning, may be a conservative exploration. I acknowledge that I can do no more that rattle the bones of the toes, which may not affect the shape of the foot, let alone alter the skeletal structure of the total organisation of society. But to challenge, even at this level, the accepted way, the taken for granted, may lead to discoveries of other possibilities, which may lead to change, or at least an awareness that the 'way things are' is not the only way things can be.

Bibliography

Albrecht, G. (1982) *The Sociology of Physical Disability and Rehabilitation* Pittsburgh: University of Pittsburgh Press
Argyle, M. (1975) *Bodily Communication* London: Methuen
Balint, M. (1975) *The Doctor, His Patient and the Illness* London: Pitman Medical Publishing Co. Ltd.
Berger, P. and Luckman, T. (1967) *The Social Construction of Reality* Middlesex: Penguin Books
Bilton, T., Bonnett, K., Jones, P., Stanworth, M., Sheard, K., and Webster, A. (1981) *Introductory Sociology* London: MacMillan
Birdwhistell, R. (1972) 'Kinesics', in T. Polhemus (ed.) *Social Aspects of the Human Body* Middlesex: Penguin Books
Boardman, J. (1964) *Greek Art* London: Thames and Hudson
Brechin, A., Liddiard, P. and Swain, J. (1981) *Handicap in a Social World* Sevenoaks: Hodder and Stoughton in association with The Open University
Bromley, I. (1976) *Tetraplegia and Paraplegia* Edinburgh: Churchill Livingstone
Campling, J. (1979) *Better Lives for Disabled Women* London: Virago
—— (ed.) (1981) *Images of Ourselves, Women with Disabilities Talking* London: Routledge and Kegan Paul
Connell, R. (1983) 'Men's bodies' *Australian Society* vol. 2, no. 9, October
Davis, A. and Horobin, G. (1977) *Medical Encounters* London: Croom Helm
Davis, F. (1963) *Passage Through Crisis* Indianapolis: Bobbs Merrill Co. Inc
—— (1964) 'Deviance disavowal: The management of strained interaction by the visibly handicapped', in *The Other Side* Perspectives on Deviance, Howard S. Becker (ed.), The Free Press of Glencoe
Douglas, M. (1970) *Natural Symbols* Middlesex: Penguin Books
Emerson, J. (1973) 'Behaviour in private places: sustaining definitions of reality in gynaecological examinations', in K. Thompson and D. Salamon (eds), *People and Organisations* The Open University. p. 358
Fabrega, H. Jnr. (1971) 'Some features of Zinacantan medical knowledge' *Ethnology* vol. X, no.1, Jan.

Folta, J. and Deck, E. (eds) (1966) *A Sociological Framework for Patient Care* New York: John Wiley and Sons

Foucault, M. (1973) *The Birth of the Clinic* London: Tavistock

Freidson, E. (1970) *Profession of Medicine, a study of the sociology of applied knowledge* New York: Harper and Row

Game, A. and Pringle, R. (1983) *Gender at Work* Sydney: Allen & Unwin

Garfinkel, H. (1962) 'Commonsense knowledge of social structures: The documentary method of interpretation', in *Theories of the Mind* Jordon M. Scher (ed.), New York: The Free Press of Glencoe, pp. 689–712

Glaser, B. and Strauss, A. (1965) *Awareness of Dying* Chicago: Aldine Publishing Co.

Goffman, E. (1959) *The Presentation of Self in Everyday Life* London: Penguin Books

—— (1961) *Encounters* Indianapolis: Bobbs Merrill Co. Inc.

—— (1968) *Asylums* Middlesex: Penguin Books

Guttman, L. (1967) 'History of the national spinal injuries centre' *Paraplegia* vol. 5, Aylesbury: Stoke Mandeville Hospital pp. 115–26

—— (1973) *Spinal Cord Injuries* Oxford: Blackwell

Handelman, D. (1975) 'Bureaucratic interpretation: the perception of child abuse in urban Newfoundland', in *Bureaucracy and World View* St. John's: Institute of Social and Economic Research, Memorial University of Newfoundland

Harrison, T. (ed.) (1962) *Principles of Internal Medicine* 4th edn, New York: McGraw Hill Co. Inc.

Hicks, N. (1979) ' The determination of policy in community health' in R. Walpole, *Community Health in Australia* Victoria: Penguin Press

Hingson, R. et al. (1981) *In Sickness and in Health, Social Dimensions of Medical Care* St. Louis: The C.V. Mosby Co.

Hirschberg, G., Lewis, L. and Vaughan, P. (1976) *Rehabilitation: A Manual for the Care of the Disabled and Elderly* 2nd edn, Philadelphia: J. B. Lippincott

Illich, I. (1976) *The Limits to Medicine* London: Martin Boyars

—— (1975) *Medical Nemesis, The Expropriation of Health* London: Marion Boyars

Illis, L., Sedgwick, E. and Glanville, H. (1982) *Rehabilitation of the Neurological Patient* London: Blackwell

Jones, H. and Jones, G. (1975) 'The resettlement process', *Paraplegia* 12, Edinburgh, pp. 251–53

Kapferer, B. (1979) *Celebration of Demons: Performance, Communication and Transformation in Sinhalese Healing Rituals* manuscript Adelaide

Kemnitzer, D. et al. (eds) (1977) *Symbolic Anthropology: a reader in the study of symbols and meanings* New York: Columbia University Press

Kleinman, A. (1980) *Patients and Healers in the Context of Culture* Berkeley: University of California Press

Kotarba, J. (1977) 'The chronic pain experience', in *Existential Sociology* J. Douglas and J. Johnson (eds), Cambridge: Cambridge University Press

Lally, J. and Preston, D. (1973) 'Antipositivist movements in contemporary sociology', *Australian and New Zealand Journal of Sociology* vol. 9, no. 2, June

Litman, T. J. (1962) 'Self conception and physical rehabilitation', in *Human Behaviour and Social Processes* A.M. Rose (ed.) (1972), London: Routledge and Kegan Paul Ltd., p. 550

Lynch, M. (1987) 'The body: thin is beautiful' *Arena* 79 Greensborough

Matthews, J. (1987) 'Building the body beautiful' *Australian Feminist Studies* no. 5, summer Adelaide

Mauss, M. (1936) (1973) 'Techniques of the human body' quoted in *Economy and Society* vol. 2, 1 February, 1973, London: Routledge and Kegan Paul pp. 70–88

McKeown, T. (1979) *The Role of Medicine* Oxford: Oxford University Press

Mead, G. H. (1934) *Mind, Self and Society* Charles W. Morris (ed.), Chicago: The University of Chicago Press

Merleau-Ponty, M. (1962) *Phenomenology and Perception* London: Routledge and Kegan Paul

—— (1964) 'The child's relations with others', in *The Primacy of Perception* J. M. Edie, (ed.) tr. W. Cobb, Evanston: North Western University Press, pp. 96–155

Mitchell, J. (1984) *What is to be Done About Illness and Health?* Middlesex: Penguin Books

Morgan, M., Calnan, M. and Manning, N. (1985) *Sociological Approaches to Health and Medicine* Kent: Croom Helm

Murrell, T. and Barker, M. (1980) *Cutting the Tripe—Paradigms about the practice of medicine in the community* Hawthorndene: Investigator Press

Natanson, M. (ed.) (1973) *Alfred Schutz Collected Papers* vol. 1, The Hague: Martinus Nijhoff

Oakley, A. (1972) *Sex, Gender and Society* London: Temple Smith

—— (1981) *Subject Women* Glasgow: Fontana

Polhemus, T. (1978) *Social Aspects of Human Body* Middlesex: Penguin Books

Richman, J. (1987) *Medicine and Health* New York: Longman

Roth, J. (1963) *Timetables: Structuring the passage of time in hospital treatment and other careers* Indianapolis: Bobbs Merrill Co. Inc.

Rothwell, R. (1984) 'The development of rehabilitation services and rehabilitation counselling in Australia 'in *Rehabilitation Counselling: Profession and Practice* J. Sheppard (ed.), Sydney: Cumberland College of Health Sciences

Russell, C. and Schofield, T. (1986) *Where it Hurts, an Introduction to Sociology for Health Workers* Sydney: Allen & Unwin

Sacks, O. (1986) *A Leg to Stand On* London: Picador

Schutz, A. and Luckman, T. (1973) tr. R. Zaner and H. Tristram Engelhardt Jnr. *The Structures of the Life World* Evanston: North Western University Press

Schutz, A. (1972) *The Phenomenology of the Social World* tr. G. Walsh and F. Lehnert, London: Heinemann

Sontag, S. (1979) *Illness as Metaphor* New York: Vintage Books

Stewart, T. (1981) 'Sex, spinal cord injury, and staff rapport' *Rehabilitation Literature* Nov.–Dec., vol. 42, Chicago, pp. 11–12

Stone, G. (1962) 'Appearance and the self', in A. Rose (ed.) *Human Behaviour and Social Processes* London: Routledge and Kegan Paul Ltd.

Strauss, A. (1963) 'The hospital and its negotiated order', in E. Friedson (ed.) *The Hospital in Modern Society* The Free Press of Glencoe

Strauss, A. et al. *Sentimental Work: A contribution to the sociology of work and occupation* manuscript, USA, undated

Strauss, A. and Glaser, B. (1975) *Chronic Illness and the Quality of Life* St. Louis: The C.V. Mosby Co.

Thomas, D. (1987) *The Experience of Handicap* London, New York: Methuen

Thorn J. and Wilbe, J. (1987) 'Rehabilitation: where are we going?' *New Doctor* 46 Paddington, pp. 7–10

Trieschmann, R. (1980) *Spinal Cord Injuries* New York: Pergamon Press

Turner, B. (1984) *The Body in Society* Oxford: Basil Blackwell

Wagner, H. (ed.) (1970) *Alfred Schulz on Phenomenology and Social Relations* Chicago: The University of Chicago Press

Westbrook et al. (1988) 'Health science students' images of disabled people',*Community Health Studies* vol. XII, Adelaide, no. 3

Young, A. (1976) 'Some implications of medical beliefs and practices for social anthropology', *American Anthropologist* vol. 78, Washington, pp. 1–2

Zola, I. (1973) 'Pathways to the doctor—from person to patient', *Social Science and Medicine* vol. 7, Oxford: Pergamon pp. 7–12

Index

ablebodied people, 102, 131
acceptance, 73, 75–6
afferent pathways, 57
age, 21–2, 30, 44, 105
alienation, 15, 61, 72, 110, 132
alternate practises, 46
alternative realities, 68, 79, 88–9, 90, 91
amputations, 3, 123
anarchy, 11–12, 15, 28–9, 124, 127
anatomy, 19, 34, 35; anatomical parts, 20
anorexia, nervosa, 18, 29
anthropology, 7, 10, 15, 22
antibiotics, 40
appearance, 97–106, 133
architectural barriers, 107
Argyle, M., 101
assimilation, 130
Ayurvedic medicine, 27–8

Balint, M., 89
barriers to transformation, 97–108
batch handling, 80
battle analogies, 61
behavioural modification, 33
Berger, P. and Luckman, T., 14, 25
Bilton, T. K., Bonnett, P., Jones, M., Stamworth, K., Sheard and Webster A., 22, 109
biology, 19, 34, 134
biomedical model, 35, 37, 39–40, 43, 49–50, 68, 71; *see also* doctors, medicine, scientific medicine
Birdwhistell, R., 108
bladder, 66, 74, 77; management, 58, 59, 60, 80, 129
Boardman, J., 11

body, 11–23; behaviour, 108; image, 6, *see also* self concept, identity, self; work, 60, 62, 64, 128, 132
bowel, 74; management, 58, 59 60, 77, 80, 129
breast, 3
Bromley, I., 57
bulimia, 18

Campling, J., 114
capitalism, 22
case construction, 69, 82
catheter, 72, 80; catheterisation, 58
childbirth, 4, 25, 38, 45, 110–12
chronic pain, 99
class, 12, 21, 30, 31, 33, 40, 44, 98, 107, 113
classificatory systems, 19–20, 34–5
clothing, 13, 22, 98, 105; *see also* dress, fashion, garments
colostomy bag, 3, 123
common sense, 8, 49, 64, 92, 132
Commonwealth Rehabilitation Service, 53
compliance, 30, 75
concept of self, 1, 2, 62; *see also* self, self concept, self identity, body image
conformity, 22, 28, 98, 126
Connell, R., 16, 26
context of meaning, 62
continuity of self concept, 122, 125, 132
control of information, 81–3, 88
cosmetics, 12, 22

data constitution, 7
Davis, F., 73, 75, 101, 104

141

death, 19, 122
deconstruction of self, 2, 66–83; *see also* depersonalisation
decubitus ulcers *see* pressure sores
deinstitutionalisation, 53
denial, 73, 75
dementia, 123
depersonalisation, 2, 66–83; *see also* deconstruction of self
deviancy, 28–9, 30, 38, 103
diagnosis, 47–51, 59, 67–71, 74
diet, 28, 31; *see also* anorexia nervosa, eating, infant feeding
disability *passim*
discharge planning, 58–9
discriminatory attitudes, *passim*; old people, 3
disease, 26, 30, 38–51; disease producing environments, 31–2, 41–2
disembodiment, 26, 46, 97, 122, 131, 132
divorce, 4
doctors, 10, 34, 59; *see also* medicine, biomedical model, scientific medicine
Douglas, M., 13
dress *see* clothing, fashion, garments
Durkheim, E., 13

eating, 17, 30; *see also* anorexia nervosa, bulimia, diet, feeding patterns, hunger, infant feeding
efferent pathways, 57
Emerson, J., 45, 79
estrangement of the body, 61, 64, 110
ethnicity, 30, 38, 40, 105
etiquette, 17
exercise, 30, 31, 32, 114–15

Fabrega, H., 36
face, expression, 100, 101; reconstruction, 3, 13, 123
fact-seeking behaviour, 76
family, 20, 21, 109, 110
fashion, 12, 98; *see also* clothing, dress, garments
feeding patterns, 18
femininity, 109, 111–15, 123, 133
fertility, 110–11

finances, 107; financial loss, 4
finite province of meaning, 84, 96, 132
food, 17, 58; *see also* eating, diet, infant feeding, feeding patterns
Foucault, M., 15, 16, 35
Freidson, E., 35

Garfinkel, H., 118
garments, 12–13; *see also* clothing, fashion, dress
gender, 16, 30, 31, 40, 44, 105, 107, 108–9; behaviour, 21, 109; and disability, 109; motherhood, 112, 115, 123; roles, 16, 109, 112; sexual relationships, 113
germs, 30, 39
gestures, 100, 105
Glaser, B. and A. Strauss, 74
Goffman, E., 68, 70, 80, 83, 86, 99, 104
grief, 2, 123
guilt, 33
Guttman, L., 56
gymnasium, 6, 62

hair, grey, 3, 133; loss, 123; style, 21
Handelman, D., 69, 82
Harrison, T., 57
health, 11, 24–37; promotion, 32–3, 42
heart disease, 2–3, 29, 49, 123, 124
Hicks, N., 34
hidden curriculum, 20
Hirschberg, G., Lewis, L., and Vaughan, P., 59
human rights, 53
humanitarian orientation, 63
humoral pathology, 27, 38
hunger, 20; *see also* eating
hydrotherapy, 6

identity, 1, 2, 62, 65, 123; *see also* self, self concept, concept of self, self image, body image
illhealth, 27–31; prevention, 31–4, 41–2
Illich, I., 42
Illis, L., Sedgwick, E., and Glanville, H., 58
independent living, 53

Index

infant feeding, 17; *see also* eating, hunger, feeding patterns
infection, 2, 4, 41, 55, 71, 72
inflammatory arthritis, 3, 124
institutionalisation, 55, 86, 128; institution without walls, 89
interpretational relevances, 116
intimacy, 110, 113, 115
intrusion of staff, 82, 88
invalid status, 133
isolation, 79

joint replacement, 3, 123
Jones, H., and Jones, G., 59

Kapferer, B., 8, 49, 50, 90, 98
Kotarba, J., 100

Lally, J., and Preston, D., 118
language, 19–20, 48, 97
legitimation, 50–1, 69
lifestyle, 30–4, 44
Litman, T. J., 74
loss of privacy, 79–82, 88
Lynch, M., 26

McKeown, T., 41
marriage, 4, 104
masculinity, 109, 114, 133
mastectomy, 3
Matthews, J., 26
maturation, 16, 18–19
Mauss, M., 13
Mean, G. H., 9, 71, 98–9
meaning province, of the patient, 49, 86, 87; *see also* specific meaning context of disease
mediators, 90–6; staff as mediators, 90–3; patients as mediators, 93–4; others as mediators, 94–6
medicine, 29, 32, 34, 36, 43, 46, 52, 54, 57; certificates, 47; medicalisation, 30; medical model of paraplegia, 67; medical model of quadriplegia, 67; rehabilitation, 52–65; *see also* biomedical model, doctors, scientific medicine
menopause, 123
menstruation, 111
Merleau-Ponty, M., 15

mid-life crisis, 123
migration, 4
mind–body–society, 23, 33 40, 60, 124, 127, 130, 132–5
Mitchell, J., 30–1
Morgan, M., Calnan, M., and Manning, N., 27, 28, 35
motherhood, 112, 123; *see also* childbirth, gender
motivation, 116; because motives, 117; in-order-to motives, 117
motor paralysis, 4
multiple realities, 84–5
Murrell, T., and Barker, M., 49
myocardial infarction, 3

Natarson, M., 8, 84, 85
National Committee of Enquiry into Compensation and Rehabilitation in Australia, 53
natural attitude, 84
naturalistic theories of illhealth, 27; humoral pathology, 27, 28; Ayurvedic medicine, 27–8; traditional Chinese medicine, 27
nature–culture dichotomy, 15–16, 19
non-verbal communication, 100–1
normality, 27–9, 38, 62, 101–2, 104, 128, 134; normalisation, 53–4, 101
nurses, 10, 57, 59, 62, 79, 80, 86, 91–2, 102, 131

Oakley, A., 109, 114
objective–subjective dichotomy, 43–5, 51, 54, 60, 62–4
occupational therapy, 6, 10, 59, 62, 78, 131

paralysis, 57, 66; paralysed limbs, 2; people, 1, 62, 74–5
paralytic poliomyelitis, 4, 55–6, 66–7, 70
paramount reality of everyday life, 84–5
paraplegia, 2, 55, 57, 64, 70–1 *passim*
participant observer, 6
Pasteur, Louis, 39

144 Bodily alterations

patient, 8–10, 60, 65, 66–96; patienthood, 99; subculture, 93–4
person, 8, 9, 60, 70, 77, 84, 93, 102
phantom limb sensations, 3
physical educators, 59
physical fitness, 26, 28, 32, 121; *see also* exercise
physiology, 19, 34
physiotherapy, 5, 6, 10, 58–9, 62, 86, 91, 131
Polhemus, T., 98, 100
posture, 18, 100–1, 105, 133
power, 33; powerlessness, 33, 132
pressure sores, 58–9, 100
psychology, 10, 32, 90
psychosocial factors, 44, 56
punk rockers, 21

quadriplegia, 2, 55, 57, 64

reconstruction of self, 2–3, 5, 84–96
rehabilitation, 3; challenge to medicine, 52–65; the dilemmas, 126–36; workers, 10, 57, 60–2, 128, 132
relevances, 47, 50, 67, 89–90, 96, 115–16, 125
religion, 16–17, 29–30
repatriation, 53; *see also* rehabilitation
reproduction, 16, 29–30, 111–12, 123; *see also* childbirth
respirator, 4, 58, 72, 81
retrospective construction of biography, 7, 118, 121, 125
Richman, J., 29
rituals, 19
Röntgen, Wilhelm Conrad, 40
Roth, J., 75, 94
Rothwell, R., 52–4
Russell, C., and Schofield, T., 34
Ryles tube, 72

Sacks, O., 18, 46
Schutz, A., 7, 35, 74, 84–5, 98, 116–17; and Luchman, T., 47–8, 50, 67, 85
scientific medicine, 40–1, 45, 89; *see also* doctors, medicine, biomedical model
selection of data, 5–7
self, 9, 60, 62, 65, 71–2, 79, 86, 89, 92, 95–7, 112, 127; self concept, 1–2, 35–6, 50–1, 65, 71–2, 123; self image, 7
sensory paralysis, 4, 57, 101, 112
sentimental work, 90–1
sex, 108; sexual function, 74, 109–12; sexuality, 16, 19, 28, 30–1, 79, 93, 107, 109–12, 133
sexually transmitted diseases, 29, 30
social action, 35–6
socialisation, 20–3; class, 23; gender, 23, 113–15; of the body, 126; primary, 79, 95; secondary, 79; within the family, 109
social phenomenology, 8, 69
social workers, 10, 59, 60, 82
sociology, 7, 10, 135
Sontag, S., 26, 49, 89
spasm, 57
specific meaning context of disease, 49–50; *see also* meaning province of the patient
sport, 56, 59, 86, 114, 118–19, 129
spinal cord, 55–7; medical management of injuries, 57; spinal injuries unit, 6, 55–9, 64, 127–8; spinal shock, 57
Stewart, T., 110–11
Stoke Mandeville Spinal Injuries Centre, 56, 59
Stone, G., 99
Strauss, A., 67, 74, 90–2
stress, 31
susceptibility to illhealth, 30, 71
symbolic interaction, 8, 97, 99
sympathy, 45, 63, 103–4, 129

taken for granted assumptions, 8, 25, 49, 84
theories, of disease causation, 27–8, 38–9, 51; humoral, 27, 38; Ayurvedic, 27–8; traditional Chinese, 27–8; individualistic, 39; germ, 39; specific aetiology, 39; monocausal, 40; multicasual 42; social, 43
Thorn, J., and Wilbe, J., 52

toilet training, 18
tracheostomy, 58, 70
transformation *passim*
trauma, 2, 4
treatment trajectory, 67–8
Trieschman, R., 58–9, 110
tuberculosis, 26–7, 41, 94
Turner, B., 14–15, 28–9, 46
typification, 10, 25–6, 35, 47–8, 50, 61, 64, 67–9, 75, 116

uncertainty, 73–9, 109, 116
unemployment, 4, 54, 112
utilitarian goals, 63

victim-blaming, 31–2
viruses, 30, 55, 64, 67, 70
vocational guidance workers, 59, 82, 121
vulnerability, 109–10

Wagner, H., 25, 47–8, 67, 74, 85, 96, 98–9, 115
Westbrook, M., 131
willpower, 89–90, 130
wheelchair, 1, 59, 74, 78, 81, 87, 100, 102, 115
women, as carers, 113; equality, 30; subordination, 16
work, 114, 129, 133; reentry, 53–4, 56, 112, 129
world wars, 53, 55, 57
wrinkling skin, 3

x-ray, 40

Young, A., 49, 68
youth, 62–3, 124, 133

zones of relevance, 25
Zola, I., 36